Savor Food,
Savor Health

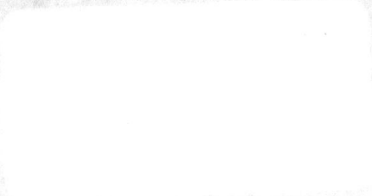

Savor Food
Savor Health

Please your palate
Overcome nagging cravings
Avoid chronic health problems
Maintain vibrant health

Carol Carpinelli

Savor Food
Savor Health:
Please your Palate, Overcome Nagging Cravings,
Avoid Chronic Disease, Maintain Vibrant Health

Copyright © 2015 by Carol Carpinelli

The content of this book is for general instruction only. Each person's physical, emotional, and spiritual condition is unique. The instruction in this book is not intended to replace or interrupt the reader's relationship with a physician or other professional. Please consult your doctor for matters pertaining to your specific health and diet.

Cover and interior photos and illustrations by shutterstock.com

Book cover design by Fatimah Bolhassan

Book typesetting by Sue Balcer / JustYourType.biz

To contact the publisher, visit
www.createhealthwithcarol.com

To contact the author, visit
www.createhealthwithcarol.com

ISBN-10:0-692-41470-3

ISBN-13: 978-0-692-41470-5

Printed in the United States of America

Table of Contents

Dedication

To my Mom and Dad, Betty and Rudy, for all your love, support and for always believing in me. You have shown me the value of family, the joy of laughter and appreciation of good food.

To Al, my life partner, for always being by my side. For every challenge we have experienced together, we keep getting stronger. I treasure you.

It is a joy and a privilege being your Mom, Andrea and Marisa. I love you more than you know. I wish continued health and happiness to you and your partners. I wish sweet baby Esmé a very bright future.

To my sisters Linda, Nancy, Karen and Chris: I value our trusted friendship and have learned a lot from each of you. We always have so much fun together.

To my extended family and friends: My life is enriched because of you.

Introduction

WE HAVE MORE CONTROL over our health than we think we do. Genetics are merely a blueprint—not our destiny. We don't have to give up the pleasure of eating delicious food. Very healthy food can also be delicious! We can enjoy good health, abundant energy, rid ourselves of nagging cravings, and avoid chronic disease by looking at the choices we are making in our daily lives that contribute to our health, good or bad.

My first introduction into health and wellness happened many years ago when my sister took me into a health food store. It was a very strange environment with many unidentified foods and products that looked foreign to me. I felt out of place and not sure I would ever go back. I didn't realize it at the time, but that visit started me on a journey that opened a whole other world to me.

Over time I began to see the connection between what I was eating, how I was living, and how good or bad my body felt. Sometime later, I began working at a health food store and loved talking to customers about the health benefits they received from changing their eating and living habits. I knew then that I wanted to help people who were struggling with ill health, low energy, and nagging cravings for junk food. That is why I work with individuals and groups as an Integrative Health Coach, so I can show those who are challenged to see a better way for themselves.

I used to be sick frequently, especially during the cold season. I suffered from bronchitis a number of times. I remember my friend saying to me, "You're sick again? You're always sick." The frustration of always being sick finally became, "Wow, I haven't been sick for a while. I think my immune system is pretty darn STRONG!"

I used to be stressed about food because I had cravings that challenged me in a way that took some of the pleasure away from just simply enjoying what I was eating. There was a time in my life when I felt out of control around desserts, and I would feel awful every time I caved in to my cravings. At that time of my life, I was stressed and not happy.

Now, I have this great sense of freedom and true pleasure in being able to enjoy food and life in general. Every day I look forward to nourishing my body and truly relishing the creative ways I can prepare food and savor a variety of deliciously prepared meals. I can go to a social gathering and not feel stressed or guilty about what I should and should not eat. That is the greatest feeling of relief and satisfaction! I have the freedom to enjoy food and know it is great fuel for my body. My motto is: Pass up the processed; eat nutrient-dense food.

Now let's journey together as I provide insight and tips on how you can free yourself from nagging cravings and enjoy tasty food that is just right for your body, whether you want to lose weight, increase your energy or are struggling with other health issues. You can choose your groceries at a health food store, grocery store or farmers market. I will show you how you can use food as medicine to create abundant energy and vibrant health for yourself.

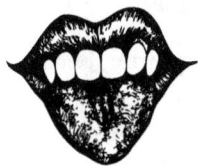

1: Reclaim Your Taste Buds

I WAS RAISED IN A FAMILY with Italian/Polish heritage. I have wonderful memories of going to my grandparents' homes as a child, especially during the holidays, gathering around a huge table with my parents, cousins, aunts, and uncles anticipating the scrumptious meal. My four sisters and I had our favorite dish—Grandma's steamy chicken soup with homemade egg noodles. The joy just poured out of Grandma as she prepared her special delicious food and watched us devour it.

Of course, my four sisters and I also ate plenty of processed food and developed a taste for it. We had our share of sugary cereals, pizza, pepperoni bread, hot dogs, lunchmeat, cookies, cakes, and powdered sugar drinks. This was and still is, the Standard American Diet or SAD.

As you will begin to see, our taste preferences from the past do not have to dictate our present appreciation of varying flavors and choices of food.

Getting to Know Our Taste Buds

Each of us has between 2,000 and 10,000 taste buds; it varies per individual. Our taste buds let us experience sweet, salty, sour, pungent, bitter, and astringent. The purpose of our taste buds is survival. They tell us whether or not to swallow what is already in our mouths. An infant is born loving sweet and hating bitter, because natural sugar is brain fuel, while bitter is the sensory cue for poison.

"The taste system evolved to protect a baby who hasn't learned anything about what is good and bad for her yet," explains Dr. Linda Bartoshuk PhD, who studies at the University of Florida, Center for Taste and Smell.[1]

According to Dr. Bartoshuk, our taste buds are constantly regenerating. They live for about ten days to two weeks, and then they are sloughed off. Your flavor preferences are not set in stone. You can train your palate to enjoy new foods.

We crave what our bodies need. Sodium is an essential mineral for muscular and nerve function; when we crave salty snacks, it might be our body's way of providing this essential mineral for itself. The type of salty food you choose, however, will impact your health in a positive or negative way. Here are some healthy options for each of your taste-bud cravings.

SALTY

- Olives
- Pickles
- Fermented vegetables (sauerkraut, kimchi, beets)
- Tabouli
- Hummus
- Oysters
- Sardines
- Salted edamame
- Sauerkraut
- Celery
- Steamed veggies with tamari
- Small amount organic cheese

SWEET

- Sweet vegetables (carrots, yams, winter squash, beets)
- Almonds
- Ricotta cheese
- Spices (fennel seed, cinnamon, cardamom, nutmeg, anise, dill, tarragon)
- Avocado
- Sesame seeds
- Sweet fruits
- Butter
- Meats

SOUR

- Yogurt
- Sour cream
- Lemons and other citrus
- Tomatoes
- Fermented vegetables (sauerkraut, kimchi, beets)
- Plums
- Raspberries
- Strawberries
- Unripe fruit (plums, pears, peaches)
- Vinegar

BITTER

- Dark green leafy vegetables (kale, spinach, collard greens, mustard greens)
- Eggplant
- Turmeric
- Chocolate
- Coffee
- Green tea
- Rhubarb

PUNGENT

- Wasabi (Japanese horseradish)
- Chilies/peppers
- Garlic
- Herbs and spices (ginger, cayenne, cloves, rosemary, cinnamon, cardamom, cumin, coriander, thyme, sage, and turmeric)
- Mustard
- Radishes
- Onion

ASTRINGENT

- Lentils
- Most beans
- Green apples
- Cabbage
- Green grapes

- Herbs and spices (thyme, nutmeg, sage, rosemary, cinnamon, coriander, basil, bay leaf, and turmeric)
- Orange and lemon peels
- Spinach
- Pears
- Rhubarb

In her book *Stop Your Cravings*, Jennifer Workman tells us:

"The primary reason the six tastes are so important is really quite simple: Variety and vivid flavors make eating more pleasurable."[2]

She explains that many Americans have forgotten this and believe that anything that tastes good must be bad for us. Many times we restrict ourselves to bland, boring food, such as a grilled chicken breast and steamed vegetables, because we believe it is the way to lose weight. In reality, we cannot stay on a restricted diet for very long. In the long run, it will cause us to crave and eat the wrong food for our bodies.

Processed Foods Hijack Our Taste Buds

Processed food has been taken from its natural form and transformed by physical means (macerating, liquefying, emulsifying) and chemical means (the long list of ingredients that you can't pronounce). The purpose of processing is to make it more appealing to the consumer with added salt, sugar, artificial flavors, and preservatives. The advantage to the food manufacturer is a long shelf life and a consumer who will continue to purchase food for artificial tastes.

Paul Stitt, a food scientist who worked for a couple of major food companies as a researcher, holds nothing back in informing the public of the dangers of processed foods in his book, *Beating the Food Giants*.

He says:

> Have you ever eaten just one Oreo cookie? Bet you can't either. They look so sweet and innocent! What you should realize is that the Nabisco Company spent millions developing that formula so that you can't eat just one. It contains 23 different appetite stimulants and 11 artificial colors. I saw the recipe and I was aghast. It's not easy to make a cookie that will hook every last American. So next time you buy a package of Oreo cookies be assured that you will eat them all at one time and gain another pound. And, the Food Giants will have another dollar in their pocket.[3]

Most of the food at the grocery store is processed, so we need to be aware of these tactics. Even if you do your shopping at a health food store, you cannot assume that everything on the shelves is healthy.

When we taste the difference between real food and processed food, our taste buds will rebel at first.

Processed food has a way of hijacking our palates, so we need to understand that there will be an adjustment period. Don't expect perfection from yourself. Keep progress in mind. Keep trying real food and notice the subtle flavors and sweetness of roasted vegetables or the cool creaminess of fruit yogurt with no added sugar. Instead of eating a donut, try:

- A piece of low-sugar fruit, such as apples, berries, pears, cherries, grapes, kiwis, plums, peaches, oranges, or nectarines. Fruit will taste sweet and satisfying after kicking your sugar habit.

- Cheese and wheat-free, low-carb crackers (buy unprocessed cheese—organic, if possible)

- Half an avocado drizzled with olive oil or lemon juice and salt and pepper
- A hard-boiled egg, lightly salted with unprocessed salt
- A handful of raw nuts
- Chopped raw vegetables, such as bell peppers, broccoli, cucumber, green beans or radishes. Dip these in hummus or guacamole for extra flavor.

Brain Connection

Researchers have found that something more complicated is going on with our sense of taste and desire for certain foods. When we eat something, for example, the taste stimuli transmit an electrically charged chemical reaction that activates a synapse in the brain and creates a communication link between cells. This is a complicated process, but it demonstrates that there are so many more factors involved in our eating habits than we may think.

The documentary, *Fed Up*, provides some great insights as to why America is facing a huge health crisis. Here are some basic points of the movie:

- There is a worldwide epidemic of obesity.
- Increased sugar consumption is responsible.
- The food industry is responsible for our increased sugar consumption because it puts hidden sugar in processed foods, bombards us with advertising, favors profits over health, and lobbies against regulation.
- The government is responsible because it has failed to control the food industry.

Two of the important messages in this movie are the following myths:

Myth 1: Calories in are balanced with calories out.

Myth 2: A calorie is a calorie, no matter the source.

What struck me when I watched this movie were the stories of the families with children, one a teenage boy and the other, a 12-year-old girl. I was saddened to see these obese young people struggle day after day with losing weight, feeling like failures because they hadn't been successful. The odds are definitely stacked against them. The majority of food available, including their school lunches, is manufactured by companies who conspire to hook people on addictive ingredients.

The majority of people believe in the first myth: Calories In and Calories Out. In other words, if you eat only the amount of calories that you burn in a day, you will not gain weight. There is the mistaken notion that if young people just get active, they will be able to lose weight, but this is not necessarily true. The movie producers stress the point: *It has to be about the food, not the calories.*

If we eat high quality food, we won't have to focus as much on the calories. Processed food with a lot of salt and chemical additives causes one to crave more sugar, more salt—more of the same. That is what the food manufacturers want; it's what they're counting on. The added chemicals and preservatives are purposeful; they make the food look and taste its best, but they also keep us coming back for more.

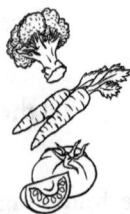

It has to be about the food—not the calories. If we are nourishing our bodies with whole, unprocessed foods, we undoubtedly will feel satisfied. We won't be constantly looking for the next sugar, salt, or chemical fix. (Think monosodium glutamate). We won't be a prisoner to our taste buds. Instead, we can make healthy choices for our bodies to satiate our cravings and our appetites.

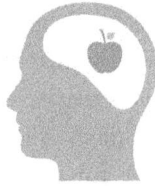

2: Overcoming Cravings

CRAVINGS ARE NOT BAD. We can learn to pay attention to our cravings.

Is there something emotional that is not being dealt with? Is the stress in your life causing you to reach for a whole bag of potato chips or a half-gallon carton of ice cream for comfort?

Our cravings can provide clues about what our body needs. If you are longing for salty snacks, you may be low in minerals. Are you restricting yourself with a low-fat diet or skipping meals to try to lose weight? The result could be counterproductive. Most likely, you will want to eat whatever is in sight without stopping.

Eat the Right Food—Eat Real Food

The first step to overcoming cravings is to eat the right foods. It can be so frustrating to get conflicting information about what foods are healthy foods and what foods we should avoid. We need to get accurate information so we can make the right choices for ourselves. This is one of the crucial things to keep in mind if you want to avoid chronic disease and have the abundant energy our bodies were meant to provide for us.

Do you ever get foggy-mind syndrome, where you know you aren't thinking clearly? Food can have a negative impact on the brain.

What we choose for breakfast to start the day will either have a positive effect on the process of our brains and bodies or it can hinder that process. Pay attention to how you feel after you eat certain foods. Does that particular food choice give you energy? Is it sustained energy or quick energy with a notable drop in your energy level? Take a candy bar or a bowl of high-carbohydrate, high-sugar cereal versus a bowl of unprocessed oatmeal with some protein like plain yogurt and chopped nuts. You will definitely get a quick boost from the processed cereal breakfast, but it will not last long. The high-carbohydrate, refined cereal will do for a short period of time, but you will soon be craving more refined carbs, sugar, or coffee to keep you going.

When you go to the grocery store, you need to know what to purchase to feed yourself and your family. What is the difference between real foods and processed foods? Real foods are foods in their natural state; a food that hasn't been stripped and broken down with added chemicals. Look for the words you can't pronounce in the ingredients list. This encompasses the large majority of foods in the store that are strategically placed at eye level and arms reach in very attractive displays.

You can choose to shop at a grocery store, farmers' market, or a health food store. There is a lot of processed food on the shelves. Be wary; look at the ingredient list and buy vegetables, fruits, whole grains, and dairy—preferably organic and grass fed, the way animals were meant to eat.

We see recommendations for various diets come and go. At this time, the gluten-free diet is popular. Not too long ago, I decided to avoid gluten, which was not a bad decision for me, but now I realize that I was seduced by many of the enticing gluten-free products on the shelves. I bought a lot of the bread, but failed to realize the cornstarch and potato starch and a few other ingredients were junk. I also had my share of the gluten-free but sugary cookies.

Many gluten free foods are high in carbohydrates and low in fiber which spikes our blood sugar and wreaks havoc on our insulin and hormonal levels. This is not a good recipe for balance and long term health.

You can buy anything gluten free now, and there are some quality foods in this category but people need to be aware that it is the next fad in the food industry. If you just replace gluten with products containing ingredients such as rice flour, sorghum flour, cornstarch etc., you will not be much better off.

Many gluten free foods are high in carbohydrates and low in fiber which spikes our blood sugar and wreaks havoc on our insulin and hormonal levels. This is not a good recipe for balance and long term health.

Gluten vs. Non Gluten

Excluding the processed gluten products I just mentioned, is it valuable for the average person to stop eating gluten even if you were not diagnosed with celiac disease? There is more and more evidence that gluten can disrupt the normal function of our bodies and cause a number of unwanted symptoms.

I have heard from many customers about the positive changes they experienced from eliminating gluten from their diets. I remember a forty-year-old woman, who had terrible acne and some gut distress, such as bloating, gas and diarrhea. She had read that people could develop sensitivity to gluten, so she thought she would try it for herself. She tried eliminating gluten for 2 weeks. After just 2 weeks she saw improvement. Over time, her acne cleared up and the gut distress was no longer an issue. Even her asthma cough that she had for twenty years disappeared!

Another case involved a younger woman, who suffered from psoriasis. Psoriasis causes red inflamed, burning, and itching skin. It is a painful condition. This woman decided to stop eating gluten and dairy. To her delight, her psoriasis vanished. She also told me that a long-time gut problem cleared up. These are cases without an official diagnosis of celiac disease, but these women decided to be proactive and try something different.

Renowned neurologist, Dr. David Perlmutter provides scientific research and his own case studies regarding the damage gluten and high-carb diets do to the brain in his book, *Grain Brain.* He talks about promoting mental stability through diet. He says that you can ward off the dreaded Alzheimer's disease by not eating gluten or having a high-carb, low-fat diet. In this groundbreaking book, Perlmutter explains what gluten does to the intestinal lining and how that can result in depression:

I encourage you to look at the evidence regarding gluten and consider what is right for you.

> A logical question: How does depression relate to a damaged intestine? Once the lining of the gut is injured by celiac disease, it is ineffective at absorbing essential nutrients, many of which keep the brain healthy, such as zinc, tryptophan, and the B vitamins.[4]

He goes on to say that a vast majority of feel-good hormones like serotonin are produced around your intestines; in fact, 80 to 90 percent of your body's requirement of this vital hormone is created there. He also clarifies that it is not necessary to have an official celiac diagnosis—a person can have gluten sensitivity and suffer the effects he describes.

Another physician, Dr. Mark Hyman who is the Director of the Cleveland Clinic Center of Functional Medicine, spends a lot of his time educating people about the root causes of many diseases. He talks about the possible causes of depression such as emotional trauma, vitamin D deficiency, vitamin B 12 deficiency, inflamed gut and an autoimmune response as a result of gluten sensitivity.

I encourage you to look at the evidence regarding gluten and consider what is right for you.

Overcoming Sugar Cravings

Dr. Bessie Jo Tillman, who graduated from the University of California Medical School, San Francisco, has a different perspective. After practicing as an emergency room doctor for 7 years and then in a walk in clinic for 3 years, as well as a private practice, she has this to say about treating people with chronic health issues:

> I loved helping people in those facilities, but I felt more could be done to prevent the suffering many patients experienced from preventable, reversible degeneration of their bodies. I began my quest for root causes of disease rather than just continuing to treat the 'end of the road' symptoms.[5]

Dr. Jo is concerned about the American diet, especially regarding sugar because it is so much a part of our daily food choices. She talks about how sugar slowly and subtly destroys the body, and often we don't even know what is happening. The cruelest part of the story is that sugar is used in such innocent ways, such as sweets and treats for children and fundraisers to raise money for schools.

> Sugar is like poison—a strong but very true statement. Not only is sugar the cause of tooth decay, as it has been known for a long time, but it plays havoc on the body in unimaginable ways.

In the last thirty years, the US rates of diabetes have nearly tripled.[6] Children are developing it at earlier and earlier ages. We also are seeing a dramatic increase in overweight people struggling with related health issues. The rates of chronic disease have continued to grow, such as high blood pressure, kidney disease, and certain cancers. Sugar also causes inflammation that can create a host of other problems like arthritis, depression, artery damage, cancer, and a weakened immune system. Some studies show that vitamin C in the body is nullified by sugar.[7]

I picked up a little book in my youth titled *Sugar Blues* by William Dufty. The information in it seemed shocking and almost unbelievable. This little book had a big impact on me. Dufty was inspired by the

Hollywood legend Gloria Swanson and wrote about the history of refined sugar and most poignantly its addictive quality and the truth of it being the greatest medical killer. He claims that a sugar-free diet can save lives.

What struck me most was his account from chronic illness to freedom and health. He began his addiction to sugar like many youth with various refined and processed concoctions that were widely available: malted milks, pastries, candy, cake with whipped cream, pie a la mode, Coca-Cola, and sugared coffee. He didn't realize it at the time, but he quickly developed a major addiction to the white stuff. Over a period of years, he suffered an unending list of maladies including: bleeding hemorrhoids, skin conditions, walking pneumonia, hepatitis, shingles, and migraine headaches. Dufty was weary from his painful headaches, lack of health, and endless medical tests and procedures. One morning he decided to throw out all the sugar in his kitchen.

> ...I threw out everything that had sugar in it, cereals, and canned fruit, soups, and bread. Since I had never really read labels carefully, I was shocked to find the shelves were soon empty; so was the refrigerator.[8]

He began eating unprocessed, non-sugared whole foods. He says that after about forty-eight hours, he was in agony with migraines, nausea and describes his experience as a difficult drug withdrawal. Dufty states that sugar is nothing but a chemical refined from the juice of the cane or beet, into strange white crystals.

He goes on:

> I was kicking all kinds of chemicals cold turkey—sugar, aspirin, cocaine, (He resorted to because it temporarily relieved excruciating headaches) caffeine, chlorine, fluorine, sodium, monosodium glutamate, and all those other multisyllabic horrors listed in fine print on the tins and boxes I had just thrown into the trash.

I had it very rough for about twenty-four hours, but the morning after was a revelation. I went to sleep with exhaustion, sweating and tremors. I woke up feeling reborn. The next few days brought a succession of wonders. My rear stopped bleeding, so did my gums. My skin began to clear up and had a totally different texture when I washed. I discovered bones in my hands and feet that had been buried under bloat. I bounced out of bed at strange hours in the early morning raring to go. My head seemed to be working again. I had no problems anymore. My shirts were too big. So were my shoes....To make a long, happy story short, I dropped from 205 pounds to a neat 135 pounds in five months and ended up with a new body, a new head, a new life.[9]

It took me a while to figure out how the sugar habit works. When I read the book, it made a lot of sense to me. At that time, I still loved pizza and pasta and my homemade cookies. I had plenty of excuses. But they were oatmeal...but they were homemade...but they still had refined sugar. I kept going back to the container that sat on my kitchen counter again and again. My whole system was set up to spike my blood sugar, not satisfy me; my blood sugar would come falling down, and I would crave another oatmeal cookie.

If you change what you eat, you don't have to worry so much about how much you eat.

If you change what you eat, you don't have to worry so much about how much you eat.

Breaking the sugar addiction may be difficult at first, but you can work through the process. If you don't think you have a sugar addiction, try going off all sugar for a week—including hidden sugars—read ingredient list on labels. It is a good idea to build yourself up first so you can better handle it.

Here is a list of things you can do to build your body up:

- Eat smaller balanced meals 5-6 per day.

- Add the good fats like omega 3's to your diet—fatty fish, flax oil, and flax meal, olive oil, grass-fed butter, walnuts.

- Eat nuts and seeds—preferably sprouted seeds for better absorption.

- Consider a whole food multi-vitamin and fish-oil or flax-oil supplement.

- Remember foods like most muffins, bread, pasta, and bagels act like sugar because they are refined.

If we stop eating refined sugar in the form of table sugar first and then slowly replace with a little raw honey, maple syrup, or stevia, we can continue to enjoy the taste of sweet. Small amounts would NOT be measured by a ½-cup or ¼-cup measurement but by the teaspoons. **A small amount as a treat occasionally is the idea.**

You might be thinking that I'm robbing you of pleasure with food. I want you to love what you are eating and savor the sweetness.

There are unending possibilities to satisfy your taste for comfort food, including the desire for sweetness.

One or two servings of fruit a day is a good way to satisfy your sugar cravings. When you start to have fruit instead of sugary foods, your taste buds will be reprogramed to appreciate the subtleness, juiciness, slight tartness, and the natural sweetness of the fruit. I love honey crisp apples! I have them as a treat. They are both juicy and crisp. Eat fruit instead of drinking

There are unending possibilities to satisfy your taste for comfort food, including the desire for sweetness.

fruit juice because the fiber in fruit is important; it's nature's way of slowing the release of sugar into your system.

Dark chocolate is also a way to satisfy the craving for sweet. If the chocolate is at least 70% cacao, it will have a small amount of sugar and still be rich and delicious. If you are not used to eating dark chocolate, try a little and see if over time your taste buds will adjust to the less sweet but creamy addition to your diet.

Dark chocolate is also a way to satisfy the craving for sweet. If the chocolate is at least 70% cacao it will have a small amount of sugar and still be rich and delicious.

In her book, *Sugar...Stop the Addiction*, Kelly Genzlinger tells us that refined sugar has no nutrients. When food comes without nutrients, it has to rob from our stores to make up for what it is missing. So if we are eating sugar, we have fewer nutrients in our bodies than we did before we ate it. Here is a list from her book of the way sugar affects our health:

- Creates mineral imbalances
- Inhibits proper enzyme function and pathways
- Disrupts hormones
- Depletes nutrients
- Inhibits proper homocysteine conversion
- Causes inflammation
- Cripples the immune system
- Predisposes food allergies
- Creates gut dysbiosis and leaky gut
- Affects attitude and perceptions
- Creates emotional instability
- Causes out of control behavior.[10]

This is not to say we should cut out all treats and deprive ourselves of the joy of eating. NOT AT ALL! We can make better choices and reap the benefits of a healthy body.

Sugar is a big deal! It is everywhere and in 80% of processed foods. No holiday, birthday party, or celebration is complete without it or so we have been conditioned to think!

This is not to say we should cut out all treats and deprive ourselves of the joy of eating. NOT AT ALL! We can make better choices and reap the benefits of a healthy body.

- If you crave something sweet, have some ripe strawberries or blueberries. Look for what is in season: melons, peaches, apples, pears. If you purchase fruit in season it will be the freshest and sweetest, especially if you buy it ripened or wait for it to ripen. The fiber in the fruit will slow the release of the natural sugar in your system, which is good for keeping blood sugar balanced.

- Find other pleasures in your life. Listen to music or watch a good movie. Play a sport you like or just move your body in a way you find enjoyable, such as bike riding, dancing or gardening. Visit a friend, take a walk in nature, try a relaxing bath, or read a book.

- There are other foods and spices that are sweet but don't have the refined sugars. Enjoy sweet potatoes, almonds, pecans, avocado, cinnamon, cardamom and nutmeg.

Refined Carbohydrates

Most of us know what refined carbohydrates are: crackers, white pasta, most breads, cakes, bagels, pizza. You get the idea. These foods turn into sugar in the body. They are devoid of nutrients, break down quickly in your system, and spike your blood sugar. Unfortunately, they are also the most widely available and sought-after foods in the American diet. Don't let anyone tell you that your body needs these kinds of carbohydrates. Just because they are on the USDA food pyramid doesn't mean we should eat them. Nutrition experts are beginning to tell us that the 5-12 servings recommended in this food pyramid may not be the best way to eat for optimal health.[11]

When I began to learn about nutrition and look at the food choices I was making for my family, I switched from white-flour pasta (my favorite food) to organic white-flour pasta and occasionally whole-wheat pasta. But now I see that really wasn't a good substitute because even whole-wheat pasta (our family would fill our whole plate with it) is very high in carbohydrates and not nutrient dense. In the long run, it does not satisfy the macronutrients our bodies need and turns to sugar, that is released into the bloodstream.

Carbohydrates like bread, pasta, bagels—that is—basically flour products—turn into sugar in the body. Eat unprocessed whole grains in small amounts. (See chapter 6.)

Crave the Good Stuff

> When we choose delicious, healthy food to nourish our bodies, the big bonus is we begin to crave the good stuff!

As I've already mentioned dark chocolate is good stuff. This tasty treat is extremely rich in a compound called polyphenols. Polyphenols are plant-based molecules that have the ability to repair damaged cells. This has the potential, as some studies have found,[12] to prevent cardiovascular disease. Scientists have also observed that the beneficial compounds in cocoa mass are able to slow the development of certain cancers, especially lung cancer induced in laboratory animals.[13]

It is possible that a craving for chocolate is a sign that our bodies are low in magnesium. Many people are low in this mineral, and chocolate is high in magnesium. Savor a piece of dark chocolate, about the size

Balance is the key. The basic macronutrients our bodies need are proteins, fats, and carbohydrates. The essential carbohydrates are vegetables, fruit, and whole grains with the emphasis on vegetables!

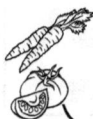

of a dental-floss container (about 2 ounces). Vegetables, such as dark leafy greens, parsley, nuts and seeds, are also high in magnesium.

I noticed the last two winters, my husband and I have been craving oranges—sweet, juicy oranges. I don't think it is a coincidence. I think our bodies instinctively knew what it is they needed—vitamin C. In the summer we are eating more fresh berries, peppers, salads, and tomatoes that are in season and are high in vitamin C. Also, winter is a drying time of year for our bodies and the heating systems in our homes contribute to that dryness. I find myself craving more liquids and juicy fruits because of it.

Balance is the key. The basic macronutrients our bodies need are proteins, fats, and carbohydrates. The essential carbohydrates are vegetables, fruit, and whole grains with the emphasis on vegetables!

Vegetables are powerhouses for our health!

Vegetables contain phytonutrients, such as carotenoids, flavonoids, and resveratrol, which are chemicals that have a therapeutic effect on the body and can help prevent disease. Vegetables are loaded with anti-oxidants, vitamin C, vitamin A, and minerals.

Let's talk anti-oxidants. We need anti-oxidants to counteract the free radicals in our cells. What are these free radicals in our cells, you may ask? Free radicals are formed because of damage to the electrons in each cell; damage can be caused by the sun, toxins, aging, and lifestyle choices. The free radicals are unpaired electrons that pillage healthy cells to stabilize themselves. This causes a chain reaction in the healthy cells, which is one thing you do not want—lots of unstable and unhealthy cells! To keep this from happening, vegetables offer anti-oxidants, which are compounds in foods that can stop free radicals from doing harm. They offer up their own electrons and prevent yours from being pillaged.

This is science—you gotta love it.

If you can understand it, you can motivate yourself to make the positive changes in your food choices and in turn improve your health and increase your chances of having a long and vibrant life! *This is the kind of chain reaction you want.*

S auté them in a tablespoon of olive oil.

S pice them with garlic, cayenne, parsley, or whatever spices you like.

S prinkle with unrefined salt.

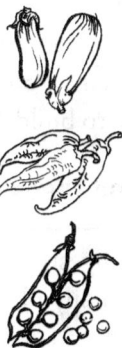

S imply add a little butter (organic is preferable). Fat will help you absorb the minerals.

S nack on them. (Cut up carrots, radishes, celery, bell peppers.)

S atisfy yourself with a freshly tossed salad.

S avor them!

Fat and Protein are Key

Balancing our food choices is important if we are to overcome cravings for food we know is not good for us. Adequate protein will help prevent us from bingeing because it will keep us full and satisfied. I will get more specific later in the book about these key nutrients. Don't underestimate the power of these winners. It is tempting to forget this fact and miss the benefits of having the right amount of fats and proteins in your life. So if you want to feel satisfied and not continually long for junk food, make sure you are having some protein and fat with every meal.

Fat is vital in keeping us satiated, because it stimulates a hormone in our bodies called leptin that gives us the signal we are full.

Fat is vital in keeping us satiated, because it stimulates a hormone in our bodies called leptin that gives us the signal we are full.

It is vital that we get enough protein and fats because not only will they help us build and maintain our muscles, organs, and nervous system, but they will also ward off the sugar cravings that can creep up on us so easily.

Balance is the key. We all need the right amount of fats, carbs, and proteins. You can learn what your particular body needs. You want to be able to build, repair, and maintain a strong body.

Good Digestion is Vital to Good Health

Digestion issues are one of the biggest health problems today. Go to any pharmacy and see how many products are on the shelves intended to relieve symptoms of gas, bloating, constipation, diarrhea, acid reflux, etc.

Overcoming digestion issues will have a huge impact on our health in a positive way; it allows our bodies to break down the food we eat and utilize the nutrients. If this does not happen in an efficient way, we will be lacking the vitamins and minerals vital to our health.

Good digestion is related to food cravings because our bodies know when there is
imbalance, and it is striving to balance itself.
The food cravings are one sign that the system is not working efficiently. Are we properly absorbing what we need from our food?

Balance is the key.
We all need the right
amount of fats, carbs,
and proteins.

Good digestion is key to good health
because the nutrients we consume affect every system and cell in our
bodies. You may have heard the claim that good digestion is 70% of
the immune system. Our digestive system has millions of good bacteria that keep the bad bacteria in check. It's a proper balance. When the
bad bacteria are allowed to overgrow, they crowd out the good guys.
They wreak havoc, weaken digestion, and produce toxins that are then
circulated in the system. This produces all kinds of negative effects,
such as food sensitivities, foggy brain, inflammation, achy joints, and
other results that we cannot even predict.

Pay attention to your body. If you have symptoms, you can make
changes that will help bring your body back in balance. Choosing the
best food is one step in the right direction.

You could also have food sensitivities; many people do. If you
think that is the case, try the elimination diet. Stop eating processed
foods including all sugar.

The common allergens are gluten (includes wheat, oat, barley, and
rye) or foods containing gluten, dairy or foods that contain dairy, eggs,
citrus and soy.

Don't eat these for two to three weeks. You have to be disciplined
and read labels. See how you feel. You may feel worse the first few days
but after that, do your symptoms subside? Put the food back in your
diet and see what happens. Introduce one of the foods, then three days
later another one and so on. Make a note of symptoms you may have.
This will give you a clue if this food is something your body cannot
handle.

One way to help replenish the good bacteria in your system, if it becomes imbalanced because of taking antibiotics or other medications, is to take a probiotic supplement. Another way is to eat fermented foods like sauerkraut, not preserved in vinegar but actually fermented. You can find this and other fermented vegetables in the refrigerator section of your health food store. Other fermented foods are available also, such as kombucha (a fermented green tea), miso, kefir and kimchi. Yogurt also has probiotics. Buy the plain yogurt; you can always add your own unsweetened fruit if you'd like.

I helped a young woman with a severe digestive problem—ulcerative colitis. This is an autoimmune disease where the immune system attacks its own tissue, in this case, the large intestine. She was under the care of a physician and her symptoms were severe. She had abdominal pain, blood in her stools, and diarrhea; she lost about 15 pounds from her already slender frame. This was her second colitis flare.

She had to be hospitalized because her symptoms were not getting any better. She needed heavy doses of steroids to reduce the inflammation and calm her overactive immune system. Even though the steroids had some very nasty side effects, this treatment lessened the severity of this attack on her body. Her doctor told her that she would always have this chronic condition; there was no cure. He explained that surgery, removing part of her colon, was the answer. She was very upset to hear this and I wanted to help her if I could. I suggested the surgery be postponed and see if her body could recover from this.

She was told numerous times that she should expect to have this condition for the rest of her life. A suggested treatment for which the doctor wrote a prescription was a chemotherapy drug intended to keep her immune system from overreacting. This drug had some severe potential side effects like making one more susceptible to infection because the immune system is dampened. The doctor said she needed to be on this medication for the rest of life, and she couldn't take it if she was pregnant.

So we had a treatment plan, which included some food elimination because I suspected she had developed sensitivities to certain foods: gluten, non-fermented dairy, and soy. She ate mostly unprocessed food and took probiotics for improving her gut flora. The idea was to cut out the junk food and eat nutrient-dense food. She continued to get better and better, and to this day she has not had another colitis flare up. That was eleven years ago. This is an extreme case, but it shows the power and ability of the body to heal itself; good digestion is absolutely vital.

Key Points to Improve Digestion and Health

- Chew your food slowly. Pay attention to the taste, take your time and chew well.

- When you first get up in the morning have a glass of warm water with fresh lemon juice. This will stimulate the digestion process.

- Eat foods high in natural enzymes, such as, raw vegetables, fruit, fermented foods (plain yogurt, miso, sauerkraut).

- Pay attention to possible food allergies or sensitivities.

- Eat smaller, more frequent meals.

- After taking antibiotics, take a probiotic supplement to replenish the loss of good bacteria from the colon.

- Eliminate refined sugar—it feeds the bad bacteria in the gut.

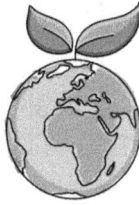

3: The Culture We Live In

A MODERN RESEARCHER and dentist took a careful look at the health and eating habits of isolated traditional societies. Weston Price travelled extensively in the 1930s and studied fourteen groups—from isolated Irish and Swiss, to Eskimos and Africans—in which almost every member of the tribe or village enjoyed superb health. They were sturdy, strong, and free of chronic disease, dental decay, and mental illness. Generation after generation, they produced healthy children. Dr. Price found that their diets contained several common factors. They ate liberal amounts of seafood or other animal protein, fats, meats, fruits, vegetables, legumes, nuts, seeds, and grains in their whole unrefined state.

It was only when these villages came in contact with western culture and the influences of western food that their health began to deteriorate. These traditional people knew what to eat and how to prepare and preserve their food for optimal health. So when we are making decisions about what is the best way to feed ourselves, it would serve us well to remember that for thousands of years, people knew how to maintain excellent health and had strong and disease-free bodies.

Pay Attention

It is crucial that we pay attention to our surroundings. We do not live separate from our culture. It affects us in ways we don't realize. Our environment includes the microcosm of our family, friends, workplace, and the greater culture outside of our homes.

> We live in an age of immense and powerful advertising. By noticing when and how we are being marketed to and how our environment affects us, we can begin to make more conscious choices about food and improve our health and quality of life.

Food, Food Everywhere

In most of our social gatherings, celebrations, and special holidays, we are surrounded by lots of food. This is one of the great joys of life! By paying attention to the quality of food we put in our bodies, we can leave our gathering feeling satisfied and nourished. You can make choices of what to eat and at the same time, not feel pressured to eat what you don't want to. This will happen when we are dining with other people, which is probably most to the time.

There can be subtle and not-so-subtle cues from others about what they want us to eat. Say, you choose not to have a piece of cake that is being served. This may be the scenario that follows (or something like it): "What!—you have to have a piece---How about a small piece?---Why not? ---Are you on a diet? ---Are you a health nut?

Maybe next time you will want to have some cake, but the point is you get to choose. We can be aware of this and understand that we alone are responsible for what we eat; we can handle the situation in a way that doesn't cause friction.

How do we enjoy ourselves at parties and celebrations, where the joy of social gathering is interconnected to the pleasure of eating what is put before us: scrumptious cookies, fancy cakes, and mouthwatering candy?

Can we still have a passion for life and a joy for pleasing our palate while partaking in healthy eating habits? YES!

Here are a few strategies to help you enjoy yourself at social gatherings and not feel deprived:

> *Can we still have a passion for life and a joy for pleasing our palate while partaking in healthy eating habits? YES!*

- Fill up on healthy food at a party: lean protein, vegetables, or salad. Enjoy something that you won't normally eat if you want, and savor it.

- Treat yourself to dessert in a small portion.

- Bring a dish or treat that you would enjoy and that has some nutrition value.

- Avoid or have a small serving of refined carbohydrates.

- Don't go to a party extremely hungry.

- If you don't buy and bring junk food into your home, an occasional splurge at a social gathering is part of being balanced and enjoying yourself.

Beware of Marketing

On our TVs are tremendous influences of marketing by giant food companies. They show us pictures of smiling, active people engaging in fun-filled activities and eating the food they produced. They tell us through their advertising of heavily sugared, chemically laden, highly processed foods that we can be these people and have these joyful experiences. However, they aren't painting a realistic future—down the road, this type of food will result in obesity, lethargy, high blood pressure, diabetes, and many chronic diseases.

Corporate and Government Involvement

Food corporations and our federal government are part of the problem instead of part of the solution for Americans. The giant food corporations have well-paid lobbyists in Washington who speak for the benefit of the food companies *not* the public.

Between the years of 1968 and 1977, a US Senate Select Committee on Nutrition and Human Needs—the McGovern committee—was in operation. Its original goal was to address the problem of hunger and malnutrition, then the issue of Americans' health regarding the rates of obesity and disease. After hearing from educators, health and nutrition experts, and school officials, the committee recommended that people should eat more fruits, vegetables, and whole grains and less high-fat meat and other unhealthy foods. The committee's "eat less" recommendations triggered strong negative reactions from the cattle, dairy, egg, and sugar industries. The American Medical Association protested as well, reflecting its long-espoused belief that people should see their doctor for individual advice rather than follow guidance for the public as a whole. Under heavy pressure, the committee issued a revised set of watered-down guidelines that didn't match the original consensus of the experts that had studied the issue.[14]

This is just one example of how we cannot assume the government and corporations have the people's best interest in mind. We must look out for ourselves and speak up for people who need to have their voices heard.

Eating Well on a Budget

The reality is it can be challenging to pay all the bills and have enough money to buy groceries. We have to eat to survive, so we have some choices to make. Having the knowledge of what it takes to provide nutritious and, of course, delicious food for our families is the first step.

Budget is a factor and so is time. You need to consider how much time you can set aside to plan, grocery shop and prepare a meal. This may seem almost impossible after working all day, but if your health depends on it (and it does), you will find a way. We will consider budget and time here because they are often both a challenge. Here are a few ideas to help you manage your grocery money and your time:

- Take the time to plan your dinners for the week ahead. Once a week, either on a Sunday or Monday, take a simple calendar and write down what you will have for dinner each day. Make a grocery list and shop once or twice a week. This is a big time saver.

- Include simple breakfasts and lunches in your planning and add to your grocery list.

- Stick to your list when you are shopping. This will save time and money.

- Simplify the process by shopping mostly the perimeter of the store; that is where the real food is and the shopping trip will be quicker.

- Don't throw away leftover food or produce. Have it for lunch the next day or make a soup or stew out of what you have in your refrigerator. Add some vegetable or chicken broth. See what spices you already have in your kitchen cabinet that appeal to you. If you have leftover meat like turkey, chicken, or beef, chop it and add it to your pot. You can also add a can of plain, basic beans to complement or replace the meat.

- Eggs are inexpensive, a complete protein, and very versatile. You can scramble them for breakfast, make egg salad for lunch, or toss them in a stir-fry.

- Buy vegetables in season for the lowest prices.

- Shop at Farmers' Markets.

- Ground meat is economical compared to other cuts.

- Look for inexpensive produce, such as cabbage, carrots, green beans, apples, celery and onions.

- Minimize the packaged food you buy. It can fool you. Some of it is cheap, and some can be expensive.

- You can get the most nutrition-dense food by careful planning and shopping. Pay attention when you shop and get more nutrients for your dollar.

Keep the planning as simple as you want.

> One idea is plan to have specific meals on certain days. For example, Monday you can cook chicken and on Tuesday, seafood or fish. Wednesday you could plan a vegetarian entrée. Repeat this plan every week. It takes the thinking out of it. Of course, you will want to vary the specific recipe of say, chicken, so it doesn't get boring.

Our Toxic Environment

There is no need to stress about the environment we live in. We can do our very best to avoid the toxins contained in beauty/personal care products, food in the form of pesticides and herbicides, and home-cleaning products.

Children and pets are more susceptible to toxic materials, so we should protect them by shielding our homes from dangerous materials. Also protect yourself and reduce the toxins that will store in the tissues of your body and potentially cause damage/weaken your immune system and cause you to store excess fat.

There are numerous products that we bring into our homes without thinking of their toxicity. Take cleaning products for example, there are hundreds of toxic cleaners in the store that we could do without.

Baking soda and vinegar are safe alternative cleaners. Sprinkle a little baking soda in your bathroom sink, and add a splash of white vinegar to a cleaning cloth. It is effective, and you can feel confident that you are not inhaling noxious fumes or having contact with chemicals against your skin. Use this same mixture for cleaning the toilet, kitchen sink, and counters (depending on the type of surface).

Dadd's message throughout the book is protecting yourself and your loved ones from toxins but-- also protecting the Earth.

There are natural cleaning products you can purchase to substitute for other toxic ones. *Nontoxic, Natural and Earthwise* by Debra Lynn Dadd contains abundant information on ways you can use simple products as substitutes. From food products, lawn and garden supplies, household pest control to baby products and energy use, Dadd provides an abundant list of helpful alternatives.

One example in this book is substituting a disinfectant with safe alternatives. According to Dadd, the harmful ingredients in disinfectants are, "cresol, phenol, ethanol, formaldehyde, ammonia, chlorine, artificial dyes, and synthetic fragrances."[15] Here are the suggestions she makes regarding replacing this toxic product:

- Clean regularly with plain soap and water. Just a hot rinse kills most bacteria.

- Keep things dry (bacteria, mildew, and mold cannot live without dampness).

- Use borax. Long recognized for its deodorizing properties, it is also a very effective disinfectant.

According to Debra Dadd, the harmful ingredients in fabric softeners are: aerosol propellants, ammonia, artificial dyes, and very strong synthetic fragrances.[16] She tells us that fabric softeners leave a residue

It is our social responsibility to take care of the environment and protect it for future generations. We are one with our environment and if the air, water and land are not clean and free from dangerous pollutants, we cannot be healthy as well.

on fabrics to control static cling that never really washes out. It can be very irritating to the skin and eyes. Try laundering without fabric softener to see if you really need to use it. To make natural-fiber fabrics softer, pour one cup of vinegar into the final rinse water. There are also natural fabric softeners you can purchase.

As far as personal-care products, it would benefit you to find chemical-free alternatives. There are many choices on the shelves, so you can also experiment and find what works for you.

- Use a little olive oil to remove make up.

- Massage some olive oil or coconut oil into your hair before washing; let it soak in from twenty minutes to a couple of hours as a conditioner. You may have to shampoo an extra time to wash it out, but it leaves your hair tangle free and conditioned.

- Use coconut oil as a body moisturizer. Rub it in your hands to melt and soften before applying.

Dadd's message throughout the book is protecting yourself and your loved ones from toxins but-- also protecting the Earth.

It is our social responsibility to take care of the environment and protect it for future generations. We are one with our environment and if the air, water and land are not clean and free from dangerous pollutants, we cannot be healthy as well.

When you are purchasing produce, it is good to know which ones are the highest in pesticides and herbicides. Depending on your budget, you can make the best choices from what is available.

The following list is from the Environmental Working Group:

The Dirty Dozen
The 12 Most Contaminated Produce

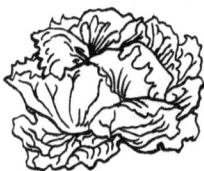
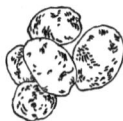

Peach	Apple
Sweet Bell Pepper	Celery
Nectarine	Strawberry
Cherry	Pear
Grape	Spinach
Lettuce	White Potato

If you are watching your budget, it's good to know that you are getting fewer pesticides in the following list of produce.

The Clean Fifteen
The 15 Least Contaminated Produce

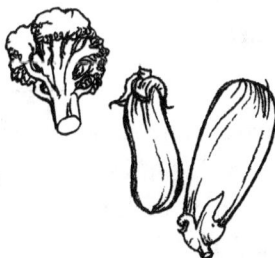

Onion	Avocado
Watermelon	Pineapple
Mango	Asparagus
Sweet peas (frozen)	Kiwi
Banana	Broccoli
Cabbage	Papaya
Sweet Potato	Cantaloupe
Eggplant	

Here are just a few suggestions to reduce the toxins in your environment:

- Don't automatically spray your lawn with weed killers. Pick some of the weeds by hand and settle for imperfection.
- Make it a habit to take your shoes off when you enter your home. Your shoes can collect toxins.
- Don't assume the beauty products you use are safe. Do some research to find out which ones are free from harmful chemicals.[17]
- Find nontoxic products to deal with pests in your garden.[18]
- Don't spray air fresheners such as Lysol and Febreze in your home.
- Use vinegar as a great cleaning product, for hard surfaces.
- Don't use plastic in the microwave.
- Use a natural body lotion with no parabens or sodium laurel sulfites, or use plain coconut oil to moisturize your skin.

So, we can see that our environment and culture have an impact on our physical health. It also affects our attitudes and priorities. Our environment affects us, and at the same time, we can have a positive impact on our environment.

We are a part of the interconnected web of life. It is about the health of our planet and everything in it—air, soil, plants, animals, lakes, streams, humans—down to each small earthworm and every microscopic insect. Our daily habits and purchases have a great impact in an accumulative way. Our health is connected to the health of Mother Earth. Let's all do our part in this—for ourselves, our neighbors, and future generations.

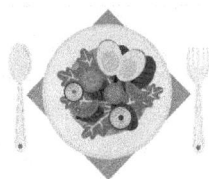

4: Stop Dieting and Start Eating

ARE YOU FRUSTRATED WITH YOUR WEIGHT and just not feeling good about what you think you should be doing? Do you get conflicting information from various sources about what is the best way to eat, what foods to avoid, and when to eat? Do you hear about different diets that make claims to help you lose weight in a specific amount of time?

What is wrong with the single-focus diet? You will not be able to keep up with this particular way of eating for very long, nor would you want to. These diets don't tell you that once you stray from the diet's narrow path, you will gain the weight back and more. Your body needs to be nourished with essential macronutrients and micronutrients.

The media is constantly putting in front of us, the quick easy fix— the answer to what program will finally work for us. But let's find a *lasting* way to eat that will help us achieve our goals of weight loss and optimum health. We generally want what is easy, but it is not always what is right for our bodies. With information about how our bodies work and the nutrition we need, we can motivate ourselves to actually follow through with a plan that will improve our lives and well-being.

Start Eating

Don't be afraid to eat. It is important to get back to finding pleasure in food. When you were a child, you had no worries about what would make you fat. You most likely thoroughly enjoyed the meal your parents put in front of you. Begin to change your perspective.

I had a client who was struggling with losing weight. We looked at her eating patterns and food choices. For her, I suggested she add a couple snack times during the day. I gave her some suggestions of healthy snacks she could eat. She likes peanut butter but always thought it was an unhealthy, fattening food, but I explained that nuts contain good fat. I encouraged her to buy the real-food peanut butter rather than the processed stuff with hydrogenated oil and sugar. She decided to cut up an apple and dip it into the peanut butter, and it was such a treat for her. She thoroughly enjoyed this new healthy snack! When I saw her at our next meeting, she was delighted to report that she was six pounds lighter.

Over the course of working with her, she saw more improvements in her weight and her health, but her greatest success was that she no longer felt controlled by her eating habits; she was now in control. She had a new perspective and delighted in the fact that she could enjoy foods that she once thought forbidden.

You might be confused about what to eat; each person is an individual with varied preferences for foods and tastes. You need to figure out what works best for your body and will nourish you effectively so you can avoid chronic disease, maintain the weight that is right for you, and keep you full of energy.

Pay Attention to Hunger Signals

Besides having a reasonable and regular eating pattern (e.g., 3 meals a day and 2 or 3 snacks a day), pay attention to your hunger signals. Your body will help you gauge how much food is too much and when it is time to eat.

If you get enough healthy fat, your body will produce a recently discovered hormone called leptin. Leptin is responsible for controlling our hunger. Nora T. Gedgaudas, an acclaimed nutritional therapist, defines leptin in her book, *Primal Body, Primal Mind*, as follows:

> Leptin essentially controls mammalian metabolism. Most people think it is the job of the thyroid, but leptin actually controls the thyroid, which regulates the rate of metabolism. Leptin oversees all energy stores. Leptin decides whether to make us hungry and store fat or burn fat. Leptin orchestrates our inflammatory response and can even control sympathetic versus parasympathetic arousal in the nervous system. If any part of your (hormonal) system is awry, including the adrenals or sex hormones, you will never have a prayer of truly resolving those issues until you have brought your leptin levels under control.[19]

When your stomach is full, fat cells release leptin to tell your brain to stop eating. It is your brake. Give your body the healthy fats it needs so your leptin signals work.

In addition, we are not used to paying attention to hunger signals. We may be working and focused and involved with a project and not think it is important. Sometimes we skip meals and think it is no big deal, but it can be very detrimental to our body rhythms and hormonal cycles. It will probably throw our eating patterns off track and cause us eat more than we need at the next meal. A good argument for always eating breakfast is that it gives us the first energy of the day and establishes a steady eating pattern. Like I said previously, aim to eat 3 meals a day and a couple snacks.

I know a few people who had great success when they applied this to their life. They thought that by skipping meals they had control over their eating and that it would result in weight loss. The opposite actually happened; the strong hunger and feelings of deprivation caused them to try to make up for the lack of food and nutrients that their bodies demanded.

Find a Flavor and Savor

Begin to experiment with different foods and flavors. There are an endless array of food preparations and spices to work with. Everyone has his own taste preferences.

I encourage you to sample different tastes that you wouldn't normally eat. Let's face it; it's easy to get stuck in a rut and eat the same few foods. What about spices? Have you tried cinnamon in bowl of whole grain oatmeal? Cinnamon has a natural sweetness to it, as does nutmeg and cardamom.

Maybe you like the sweetness of coconut; try sprinkling it on your next serving of yogurt or oatmeal. You can also buy shredded coconut and coconut flakes. They have a nice, chewy texture. Buy the unsweetened ones. You can toast it to give it a little different taste variation:

Spread it out on a cookie sheet and toast in a 375-degree oven until golden (about 10 minutes) Try making your own parfait by layering yogurt, fresh fruit, coconut, and maybe some chopped nuts. Use whatever ingredients appeals to you. This is refreshing in the summertime.

Try out vegetables that you wouldn't normally eat. Bake a sweet potato to the perfect doneness. It is so smooth and a little sweet. It's great with a pat of butter added. How about brussel sprouts? They are great sautéed with some olive oil, or butter, sprinkled with garlic and maybe a hard cheese, like parmesan.

I just discovered that I like spaghetti squash. I cut it in half length-wise and scooped out the seeds and put it cut side down in a pan with about an inch of water. It took about 45 minutes to bake in a 375-degree oven. I let it cool and then scooped out the flesh. I flavored it up by melting a couple of tablespoons of butter in a fry pan. (Remember butter is good.) I then add about 2 tablespoons of chopped soft herbs. You could use parsley, basil, chives, sage, or a combination of a couple. I added some salt and pepper to taste. Then I added the spaghetti squash to this mixture in the pan and heated it and gently stirred. I thought it was delicious. I was looking for a snack and actually ate this cold the next day.

> Eating pleasure is about appreciating all the different flavors and textures that food has to offer. In the summer, ripe berries are so good. They are plump and juicy, and you just want to pop them in your mouth.

Have you tried making a pudding with healthy ingredients? Here is a recipe for chocolate pudding with avocado. It is so creamy and good with the great benefits and the fat of the avocado.

Chocolate Pudding
Serves 3 to 4
Note: This is a rich pudding, so a small serving is satisfying.

3 avocados
¼ cup honey
6 tablespoons raw cacao powder
1 teaspoon vanilla
¼ teaspoon sea salt
Milk, almond milk or other milk substitute, as needed

Place the ingredients in a blender or food processor and process until creamy. While blending, add some water, milk or almond milk, a teaspoon at a time if it is too thick. Enjoy!

I have recently discovered the joy of Indian spices. I have always liked Indian food but now appreciate the flavors and spices even more. A few Indian friends have cooked for me, and I just love the pungent and savory spices of cumin, mustard seed, coriander, turmeric, and of course garlic. I am just starting to experiment with cooking with these wonderful flavors.

It's great to cook at home, but sometimes we want to go to a restaurant. This is a great opportunity to try new and different foods and find out what you like.

A few suggestions for restaurants where it is easier to make healthy choices: Greek, Middle Eastern, and Asian. They tend to include more vegetables in their dishes, use simple unprocessed ingredients and the food is cooked using a healthier method.

If You Love to Eat, Motivate Yourself to Cook

It is important to cook the majority of your meals in order to eat healthy. I really don't see how to get around it. When we cook for ourselves we get to control the quality of the food and best preparation method. It takes a little time to do some food preparation, for example, to wash some lettuce greens and chop some vegetables for a crisp, fresh salad. It does take some time and planning.

With the right kind of planning and just a little creativity, cooking doesn't have to be a burden.

With the right kind of planning and just a little creativity, cooking doesn't have to be a burden.

You might be saying to yourself that you are too busy to cook or you aren't interested in cooking. Again, keep it simple and keep telling yourself you are making a positive effort to get healthy and stay healthy. There are many ways you can make it work. You can cook when you have a little time and freeze or refriger-ate or you can plan to make a double

Your LIFE depends on the fact that you can provide tasty, quality food for yourself.

batch of something and eat it more than once. If you still doubt that you can perform this task think about if you have a task at work that you don't like doing but you know you will get it done because your job depends on it.

Your LIFE depends on the fact that you can provide tasty, quality food for yourself.

I spend some time in the kitchen every week, but I don't mind cooking and I choose simple to more complicated recipes depending on how much time I have and what I feel like preparing. I figure it takes time driving to a restaurant, waiting for a table and your food and get-ting back home. Cooking is worth the time put into it. I don't mind cooking because I like to eat delicious, nutritious food!

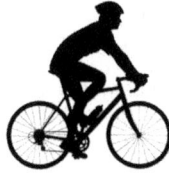

5: Beyond Food

Stress

> Unfortunately, we can't avoid stress; it is a part of living. We all have responsibilities and day-to-day details, such as getting to work on time, paying our bills, taking care of children and loved ones, buying food, preparing food, etc. We can learn to recognize how it affects us and learn to reduce it.

You may not recognize how stress is affecting you. It could be in the form of tension in the body: tight shoulder muscles, holding muscles in the forehead and neck that could cause a headache, sitting too long and getting a lower back ache. Begin to see how you deal with stress and if you work with it in a positive or negative way. Stress and tension can show up in our relationships and cause us to be impatient or unreasonable with our loved ones or our coworkers, for example.

When we crave unhealthy food, it can be because we are not taking care of ourselves and not dealing with stress in a healthy way. What we need to do is take really great care of ourselves in the way that is right for us. One effective way to deal with stress is to move our bodies.

Get Moving, Keep Moving

Exercise plays a key role in health in general and in reducing stress. You are starting to say to yourself, "I know I need to exercise. It is good for me, it will help me lose weight, be healthier, and reduce my blood pressure." Listen to your inner wisdom. There are so many ways that you can find to move your body and feel good in the process. Lose the excuses. Notice how exercise releases tension. The most important message here is to just MOVE!

Find what works for you. What do you enjoy doing? Do you like to play a sport? Do you enjoy running, gardening, walking, biking, kayaking or skiing?

I have learned to enjoy moving my body and move it in many ways. I still need to look for opportunities to do so because I can let a busy schedule get in my way. I will stop what I am doing, if I am working at the computer, for example, and stand up and stretch. I will break into a yoga pose like mountain pose, cat and cow stretch, and my favorite, downward dog. In this position, you end up folded in an upside down V with your arms extended and feet on the ground. Downward dog releases tension in the shoulders, stretches the hamstrings, increases flexibility in the Achilles tendons, and aligns the spinal column. I tend to carry tension in my shoulders, and I can tell it is being released with this position.

Yoga is great for improving flexibility, strengthening muscles, and reducing stress. Yoga also helps you be more conscious of your breathing and use your breath as a way to be aware of what's going on in your body and reduce stress. I tend to take short quick breaths when I am overtired or feeling some stress. If I consciously slow down and take deep breaths, I can feel myself begin to relax.

When we exercise, we may often feel that it is drudgery, but that doesn't have to be the case. A good book, *Sitting Kills, Moving Heals*, written by the former director of NASA Life Science Division, Joan Vernikos tells us how. Joan says that paying attention to our everyday movements is the foundation for a sustainable exercise plan. She tells us that being creative and using gravity to our advantage can help us have a strong, fit body.

We can remember what it was like to move our bodies when we were children and have fun, whether we like bike riding, dancing, skiing, or gliding on swings at a playground. I did try the swing at a nearby playground and enjoyed it.

Through her research in working with astronauts, Ms. Vernikos details the effects of a lack of gravity:

- Heart shrinkage
- Loss of muscle mass
- Blood volume reduction
- Muscles less able to take up sugar
- Increased fatigue
- Aching joints
- Disturbed sleep

This is just to name a few. This lack of gravity equates to our sedentary lifestyles. She says that our gravity habits or G-habits are what matter. Many of us spend long periods of time at our computers, so standing often will exert your G-force and help prevent the physiologic changes induced by a sedentary lifestyle. Just as astronauts' bodies forget how to live in gravity, our bodies will also.

Don't think of exercise as a chore; think of it as a way to reduce stress, feel good, build a strong body, and extend your life at the same time.

As I was working at the computer one afternoon, I paid attention to my G-habits. I noticed how often I got up to fix myself a cup of tea, to retrieve something from another room, or to get to the phone. I would also stop what I was doing and stand up. I counted how many times I stood up from a seated position and was surprised to find out that I put my body in motion 42 times. Joan Vernikos's research tells us that it is not how long one stands but how often you move your body to a standing position that matters.

Don't think of exercise as a chore; think of it as a way to reduce stress, feel good, build a strong body, and extend your life at the same time.

Emotional Eating

I experienced emotional eating when I was younger, and it's a very uncomfortable feeling. Trying to fill up with food to deal with stress or emotions is detrimental to our health. Recognizing our emotions and trying to understand them is a productive thing to do. Sometimes we are not able to deal with our emotions ourselves, and we need to seek out professional help.

We may overeat because of boredom, loneliness, or stress. When we let stress build up without dealing with it, it can intensify and cause feelings and behavior that are difficult to deal with. Stress reduction will definitely help with emotional eating.

Depression

Many people suffer depression from mild to severe. There are many causes of depression from emotional trauma, environmental causes, loss of loved ones, and perceived loss of control of one's life. There can also be a lack of vital nutrients that the brain needs to function to its capacity. Our brain chemicals such as dopamine, endorphins, norepinephrine, and serotonin play a crucial role in our wellness. If serotonin is in short supply, depression as well as insomnia and food cravings may result. High levels of serotonin, for example, can impart feelings of calm and wellness. Low levels of endorphins—the feel good chemical—cause us to feel overwhelmed and emotionally unstable because our neurotransmitters can't function properly without protein, fats, vitamins, and minerals. Research has shown that a number of nutrients—B vitamins, vitamin C, and selenium—convert amino acids in our diet to mood-lifting neurotransmitters.

Fat is crucial for the brain. Omega 3 fatty acids, as found in fish, provide great benefits. Lorna R. Vanderhaeghe and Karlene Karst, authors of *Healthy Fats for Life* have found in their research that countries with higher fish consumption have lower rates of depression and bipolar disorder.

In her book *Sugar...Stop the Addiction*, Kelly Genzlinger, explains the roller coaster ride that results from eating a diet high in refined carbohydrates and sugar and low protein and fat. Here is her break down of optimal blood sugar characteristics vs. low-blood sugar characteristics:

Optimal Blood Sugar	Low Blood Sugar
Energized	Exhausted
Tired at night, appropriately	Not enough energy
Sharp Mentally	Foggy Mentally
Relaxed, but engaged	Restless, keyed up
Good memory	Poor memory and concentration
Calm, steady	Irrational bursts of anger
Even-keeled temperament	Frustrated (too easily) [20]

Joy

I believe the purpose of life is to be happy. Of course we can't forget about other people in that happiness. In fact, when we show compassion to others and do what we can to help them, we find that it comes back to us. Finding joy will contribute to your well-being and positively affect your health.

What makes you happy? Is it watching a brilliant sunrise or sunset? Is it playing with a child? Is it cooking for others? Is it moving your body, or playing a sport? Is it studying and improving yourself? What about enjoying delectable food? What makes you feel good? Being with friends and family? Do you feel joy sitting on a beautiful beach in the sunshine?

Find what brings you joy—savor it—and share it with others!

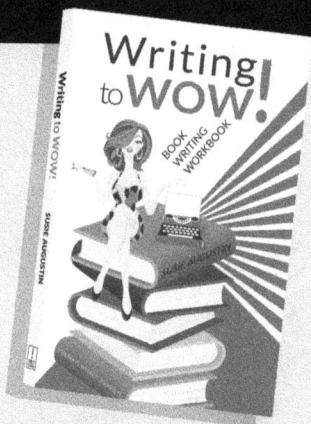

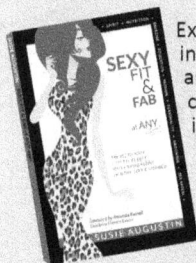

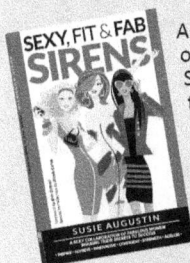

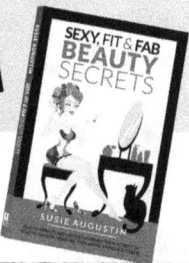

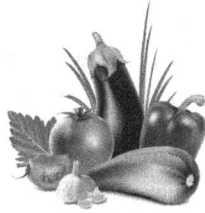

6: *The Benefits of Real and Delicious Food*

UNTIL RECENTLY, FAT HAS BEEN vilified as the worst possible thing for our health.

We have been hearing for a number of years that fish and fish oil is beneficial, but as far as other fats, we have been told they are not necessary in our diets. It is a mistaken notion that fat in food makes us fat.

The major food companies back in the 1970s started taking the fat out of food and adding sugar. We were told that science points to fat in our food as the cause of the increase in weight gain in Americans. Many products on the shelves boasted NO FAT or LOW FAT. But now a number of researchers and physicians are challenging the old facts and coming up with new information that is debunking the old data.

Fat is Good, Fat is Back

Within the different types of fat are the omega-3 fats that fish contains. This is the category of:

Polyunsaturated fats. There is omega 3 fats in deep water fish such as salmon, tuna, halibut and sardines. You can get it from fish oil, flax

Until recently, fat has been vilified as the worst possible thing for our health.

On the other hand, fat is what makes food taste great and we shouldn't be afraid of it—the good fat.

seeds, and walnuts. We want to get adequate omega 3-oils; most people do not.

Monounsaturated fats tend to be liquid at room temperature and solid when refrigerated. Examples of monounsaturated fats include: olive, avocado, and sesame.

Saturated fats are found in animal foods and tropical oils, such as coconut and palm oils.

Trans fat or hydrogenated fats are the bad guys. Trans fat is found in processed or junk food, such as baked goods, French fries, and doughnuts-- check labels.We should avoid these types of foods or have them only on rare occasions.

The purpose of hydrogenating fat is to extend its shelf life. You want to extend *your* shelf life—so don't eat it!

Trans fat is artificially produced, and it is identified on food labels as hydrogenated or partially hydrogenated oils. This type of fat increases inflammation and decreases HDL, the good cholesterol, which boosts your risk for heart disease.

On the other hand, fat is what makes food taste great and we shouldn't be afraid of it—the good fat.

I was influenced by the general consensus that fat would make us fat and fat would clog our arteries. I remember steering clear of it at all costs. It was nasty stuff, and I would not want something that bad to cross my lips and be ingested in my system. I had to eat something and carbohydrates seemed like the best thing to eat. I ate plenty of bread, pasta, pizza, oatmeal cookies, crackers, etc. I didn't have a weight problem, but I was sick a lot with colds, the flu, and bronchitis. Now that I have introduced the good fats back into my diet and reduced many of the refined carbs, I notice that my immune system is much stronger than it has ever been. That makes me very happy. Nobody likes to be down with a bug.

I have a 39-year-old friend, who struggled with respiratory problems since he was a child. He had asthma, frequent colds, and developed pneumonia every winter. The severity of his condition would, at times, get in the way of him being able to function to his full capacity in a given day.

He decided to change the foods he was eating, mainly by increasing the fats in his diet significantly. He enjoyed grass-fed butter, coconut oil, and olive oil. He cleaned up his diet, made sure he got adequate protein, and cut out most of the sugar and carbohydrate grains (bread, noodles, rice, etc.). Amazingly, he is enjoying a dramatic change in his health with no asthma attacks, colds, or pneumonia infections. He has not had to use his inhaler for over a year, and previously he had to use it on average 5 to 7 times a week, sometimes more. He lost 30 pounds and went back to his high school weight of 145 pounds. Another great benefit is that his cholesterol levels went down significantly.

Saturated Fat is Not the Enemy

For the last sixty years, saturated fat has been deemed the enemy. How did this happen and why are new researchers and some doctors challenging this theory?

In the 1940s, Ancel Keys began the Seven Country Study, which looked at the dietary habits of businessmen in seven countries. His conclusion was that dietary fat—specifically saturated fat—was the culprit in the increased incidence of coronary heart disease.[21] The study reference is called the diet lipid theory. Keys presented his conclusion in 1970. From that time on, health professionals recommended a low-fat diet and elimination of saturated fat.

This theory has been questioned by a number of researchers and doctors. Cardiologist Aseem Malhotra wrote an article in the *British Medical Journal* challenging Key's conclusion. The study failed to include other vital risk factors such as smoking rates, sugar consumption, and exercise levels. Also twenty-two countries were a part of the study, but Keys zeroed in on only seven excluding the remaining communities, such as Kenyan, Masai, the Tokelau in Polynesia, and the Artic Inuit, from the final report.

Admittedly, this theory of dietary fats and heart disease can be a complicated one; including total cholesterol levels are not as important as your ratio of triglyceride level (LDL) the bad cholesterol, and your high-density lipoprotein (HDL), or good cholesterol.

In the past thirty years in the United States, according to the *British Medical Journal,* the amount of calories from consumed fat has fallen from 40 percent to 30 percent, while obesity has doubled and heart disease has remained the country's number one killer.[22] Food manufacturers gladly heeded the low-fat call to action in the 1970s and removed and reduced fats from their products; however, if you look at labels, you will see the large amount of sugar that has replaced the fat. It is up to us to draw our own conclusions on what is the right way to eat for a healthy heart and strong body.

In the 1960s, data collected from research on coconut oil was misinterpreted regarding its effect on our health. Experts in the field of fats and oils show that coconut oil is rich in lauric acid, a proven anti-viral, anti-bacterial, and anti-fungal. Coconut oil will actually speed up the metabolism so its benefits could also include weight loss.

This is what Dr. Joseph Mercola, an osteopathic physician, has to say about saturated fat:[23]

Saturated fat plays a key role in cardiovascular health. The addition of saturated fat to the diet reduces the levels of a substance called lipoprotein that correlates strongly with risk for heart disease.

1. Stronger bones. Saturated fat is required for calcium to be effectively incorporated into bone. According to one of the foremost research experts in dietary fats and human health, Dr. Mary Enig, Ph.D., there's a case to be made for having it be as much as 50 percent of the fats in your diet for this reason.

2. Improved liver health. Saturated fat has been shown to protect the liver from alcohol and medications, including acetaminophen and other drugs commonly used for pain and arthritis.

3. Healthy lungs. For proper function, the airspaces of the lungs

have to be coated with a thin layer of lung surfactant. The fat content of lung surfactant is 100 percent saturated fatty acids. Replacement of these critical fats by other types of fat makes faulty surfactant and potentially causes breathing difficulties.

4. Healthy brain. Your brain is mainly made of fat and cholesterol. The lion's share of the fatty acids in the brain is actually saturated. A diet that skimps on healthy saturated fats robs the brain of the raw materials it needs to function optimally.

5. Proper nerve signaling. Certain saturated fats, particularly those found in butter, lard, coconut oil, and palm oil, function directly as signaling messengers that influence metabolism, including such critical jobs as the appropriate release of insulin.

Note: Cholesterol, which is made from saturated fat, has benefits that some researchers are now noting. It plays an important role in building cell membranes, interacting with proteins inside your cells, and helping protein pathways required for cell signaling. Having too little cholesterol may negatively impact your brain, hormones, and heart disease risk.

6. Strong immune system. Saturated fats found in butter and coconut oil (myristic acid and lauric acid) play key roles in immune health. Loss of sufficient saturated fatty acids in white blood cells hampers their ability to recognize and destroy foreign invaders, such as viruses, bacteria, and fungi.

Fats and oil experts, such as Mary Enig, believe butter is better and should not be replaced with hydrogenated fats like margarine and other butter substitutes. For a lean and healthy body, enjoy butter!

Lorna R. Vanderhaeghe and Karlene Karst, authors of *Healthy Fats for Life* explain:

> Butter contains many healthful components, including lecithin, which aids the body to break down cholesterol. It is also a rich source of vitamin A, which is necessary for the healthy functioning of the adrenal and thyroid glands. The vitamin A and E and the mineral selenium in butter also serve as important anti-oxidants in protecting against free radical damage that can destroy tissues and weaken artery walls.[24]

Enjoy some butter

The authors go on to tell us that butter contains conjugated linoleic acid or CLA, an essential fatty acid. It was first discovered in the 1930s and considered to be necessary for both cell growth and as a building block for cell membranes. CLA occurs naturally in dairy foods and grass-fed beef and lamb. The content of this vital nutrient has declined over the last several decades due to the increased antibiotic use in cattle and change in the way they are fed. Instead of feeding them the way nature intended, they are artificially fed with large amounts of grains.

If your budget allows, buy grass-fed butter, dairy, and meat.

There are over 500 published research studies supporting CLA's positive benefits including fat loss, prevention and control of type 2 diabetes, protection against heart disease, and keeping the immune system functioning properly. It may also inhibit the growth of certain kinds of cancers, such as breast, prostate, and colon. Eating saturated fat in the form of eggs, yogurt, poultry, and meat is not going to harm you; in fact, it will give you the B vitamins, zinc, and iron that you need to function.

Some, for ethical reasons, may not want to eat animals or their products. There is a huge difference between factory farms or industrial farms and small, local farms. I know that the animals on industrial farms, where most of our meat is raised, have horrible conditions. If you choose a small, local farm, however, the animals will not be subjected to the conditions that mass production exposes them to. The animals will be healthier, and therefore, the meat and dairy will be also. The environment will not be polluted like it is from large industrial farms because of all the pesticides and chemicals.

If you still are against eating meat, consider having some dairy products like eggs and cheese. It is difficult to get all the nutrients and digestible protein from vegetable sources.

H. Leon Abrams puts it this way in his book, *Vegetarianism: An Anthropological/Nutritional Evaluation*:

> No culture in the history of mankind has been based on a one hundred percent vegetarian diet, and although one can theoretically, in the light of contemporary nutritional scientific knowledge, obtain all the nutrients needed to provide good health, the technology to insure such has not been developed and such a vegetarian diet is extremely risky.[25]

A client I helped with overeating and weight gain was delighted to hear that she didn't have to feel guilty about choosing to eat some cheese for a snack; she saw weight-loss results because the fat and protein in the cheese satiated her and helped with her cravings.

Besides giving our food its wonderful texture and flavor, fat provides numerous benefits for our health. Here are a few of them:

- Helps our brain function properly. (Our brains are 60% fat.)
- Stimulates the production of the hormone leptin, which tells us when we are full.
- Natural fats help us absorb fat-soluble nutrients, such as, EADK and CoQ10.

Here are a few suggestions of healthy foods with fat to get you started, so you can feel confident that they are benefiting your health:

- Avocado (Drizzled with lemon juice and a little salt.)
- A handful of walnuts, pecans, or almonds
- ¼ cup of pumpkin seeds or sunflower seeds
- Full fat dairy, such as yogurt, cheese or kefir

Increase the good fats in your daily food plan because if you are on a low-fat diet, you will invariably reach for the carbs.

Carbs, Carbs Everywhere

Carbs—we just love them! We love our pastas, our garlic bread, our big fluffy sandwiches, our stuffed pizza, our crispy crackers, our salty chips, our delightfully sweet and chewy cookies, our moist chocolate cakes, and our bubbly Cola drinks.

> Carbs are everywhere we are—parties, the work lunchroom, the birthday party, our schools, and in every grocery store aisle. We want them, and we long for them for so many reasons, but what is wrong with them? Do we really need them to survive?

They are actually ruining our health. That is a strong statement, but it is true.

I grew up with all this stuff, so I feel a little guilty trashing it. What, you might be asking, is so bad about carbs? After all, everyone eats this way, and you probably haven't seen anyone drop dead after consuming them.

The truth is carbs are empty calories with little nutritional value. They make us crave more and more and make us feel sluggish. We don't see what effect they have inside our bodies.

I can say that after making a change in the way I look at food and took the steps I needed to take; I feel 100% better! I didn't realize that I wasn't feeling my best. I felt fatigued and sometimes exhausted. I also had foggy brain. I thought this was a normal way to feel. I told myself I was tired because I had a busy life. Also, I had cravings for food that I knew wasn't good for me, but was too frustrated to do anything about. My stomach was frequently bloated but I carried on and if I hadn't begun to realize over time what I needed to do for myself, I would still be settling for a less than quality state of health.

> The truth is carbs are empty calories with little nutritional value. They make us crave more and more and make us feel sluggish. We don't see what effect they have inside our bodies.

I am very grateful that I have the knowledge and the motivation to make the right food choices for myself. You can do the same and have the best quality of life possible!

Whole Grains

Whole grains contain all the essential parts of the grain seed or kernel, which includes the bran, the endosperm and the germ. In processing, the grain is stripped of the bran, which is the outer layer. The bran contains a lot of necessary fiber and nutrients such as vitamin E, B vitamins and many important minerals. These nutrients are discarded in the refining process.

Some examples of whole grains are:

- Buckwheat
- Quinoa

- Rice –both brown and colored
- Millet
- Rye
- Wheat
- Oats –rolled oats and steel cut oats

Millions of people can't properly digest gluten and must choose gluten-free grains such as:

- Teff
- Amaranth
- Rice –both brown and colored
- Sorghum
- Wild rice
- Buckwheat
- Oats

Note: Oats are inherently gluten free but are frequently contaminated with wheat during growing and processing. Look for gluten-free oatmeal if you think you have gluten sensitivity.

Benefits of No Grain or Low Grain

People with digestive issues and other chronic health issues should consider cutting out grains in their diet, at least for a short period of time—3 weeks. See how your body reacts to it. Reducing grains, even if they are whole grains, can definitely benefit you.

Our bodies were not meant to digest grains. Also, grains will stimulate an insulin response, which results in a cascade of your hormonal responses, raising cortisol levels, which in turn gives the signal to your body to store fat. When your cortisol levels drop, your body will try to get back in balance and the hunger drive will kick in and cause you to eat more in order to raise the blood sugar. As you can see, it is a bumpy roller coaster ride, instead of calm, smooth sailing. This rise and fall of blood sugar and hormonal levels is connected to our brains, so it could also affect mood, stress and mental clarity.

If you decide to eliminate all grains, know that just like the initial withdrawal period from sugar, the first several days may be challenging. You may experience some unpleasant symptoms of nausea, headache, fatigue and general malaise. It won't last forever, just for those first four or five days.

The benefits will last a lifetime!

Powerful Protein

Protein packs a punch! It contains the amino acids that are the building blocks for our cells. Many people don't get enough protein in a day. We should make sure to get it at every meal.

If you are struggling with weight and health issues, include it in every snack also. It is difficult to get enough digestible protein when you are a vegetarian but not as difficult if you choose to eat eggs and dairy. Protein will make you feel full and satisfied. It is the anti-diabetes food. I find that if a person is not getting enough protein, they most likely, will be filling that void with sugary, starchy carbs. This is the worst thing for us!

Keeping our blood sugar at an even level is so important to prevent diabetes and many chronic diseases such as heart disease and depression.

Having a consistent blood-sugar level will make a world of difference in these areas:

Protein packs a punch! It contains the amino acids that are the building blocks for our cells. Many people don't get enough protein in a day. We should make sure to get it at every meal.

• Reduces the occurrence of Alzheimer's disease[26]

- Keeps blood cholesterol level in range
- Controls anxiety
- Aids in better sleep
- Reduces cancer risk. (Cancer cells feed on sugar and refined carbohydrates.)

These are big claims, but we can't underestimate the importance of having normal blood sugar levels and what a serious consequence there is for our health if we don't.

There are lots of ways to work protein into your meals and snacks. Be creative and ENJOY!

There is new evidence that our blood cholesterol levels are influenced mostly by the refined carbohydrates we eat and not the saturated fat. Elevated triglycerides in the blood have been positively linked to proneness to heart disease but some researchers say it is caused by the consumption of refined sugar and white flour. Again, refined carbohydrates are processed grain such as: crackers, bread, pastries, cookies, pasta, noodles and rice.

So we see the importance of getting enough protein as a start in balancing our macronutrients for better health and disease prevention.

Here are some suggestions for protein rich foods:

- Eggs
- Cheese (preferably organic)
- Beans
- Handful of nuts
- Poultry (chicken or turkey—preferably pasture raised)
- Yogurt (no added sugar)
- Beef (grass fed—not industrial farmed)

There are lots of ways to work protein into your meals and snacks. Be creative and ENJOY!

Many Herbs and Spices—Many Benefits

Sweet, spicy, pungent, bitter—there is an abundance of herbs and spices to satisfy your unique tastes; they can satisfy your taste for sweet, wake you up, stimulate your endorphins, give you a boost of energy, and aid in an endless number of ailments. The best part is there are NO SIDE EFFECTS.

In her book, *Nourishing Traditions*, Sally Fallon shares what Claude Aubert, an agricultural engineer and promoter of healthy food, says about how spices can aid in digestion:

The first phase of digestion begins in the mouth where the enzyme, amylase becomes mixed with the food we are chewing and begins to digest starches. The production of saliva… [is] stimulated by several spices, notably pepper, ginger, hot pepper, curry and mustard. Research shows…that these spices and condiments can increase their activity (of saliva and enzyme production) by as much as 20 times.[27]

Many herbs and spices have **anti-oxidant properties**, which mean they work on a cellular level in the body to counteract the oxidation from free radicals that come from aging, sun damage, stress, and poor-eating habits. Some of those herbs include:

- Ginger
- Celery

- Green tea
- Milk thistle
- Rosemary
- Turmeric

Here are some herbs and spices that **aid digestion**:

- Anise
- Cinnamon
- Chamomile
- Ginger
- Rosemary

If you are looking to **reduce your chances of getting a cold or flu**, try these herbs and spices:

Garlic
Ginseng
Green tea
Ginger
Turmeric
Maitake and shiitake mushrooms (though these aren't technically spices)

Try **stimulating endorphins, the feel good chemical**, by eating:

- Chilies
- Cayenne pepper spice

Decrease your chance for developing cancer and also **inhibiting cancer growth** with these herbs and spices:

- Ginger
- Licorice
- Green tea
- Turmeric
- Orange and lemon peel
- Rosemary
- Parsley
- Cloves
- Basil
- Thyme

I love the taste of cinnamon so I like to hear that it has healing properties. Cinnamon has anti-oxidant properties and is great for helping the body process sugar more effectively. Many people can benefit from putting this spice in oatmeal, sweet potatoes, coffee or whatever you like because it stimulates insulin activity.

I also like garlic a lot and grew up eating a good amount of it, but have to be careful because those around me may not like it as much. Sally Fallon says this about garlic:

> ...garlic and onions have long been valued for their use in cooking, as pickled snacks and for medicinal purposes. Studies have corroborated the belief that these foods hinder the growth of intestinal parasites and germs and help fight off infections, both in the digestive tract and in the lungs. Garlic, and to a lesser extent onions, are rich dietary sources of sulphur and selenium. The

traditional use of garlic for the prevention of blood clots also has recently been corroborated by science. Researchers have identified a substance called adenosine in garlic oil that breaks down a blood-clot promoting protein called fibrin.[28]

Turmeric is an amazing medicinal spice. It gives Indian food its flavor and wonderful bright yellow color. The principle compound in turmeric is curcumin. The Chinese and Japanese use this spice therapeutically as it has a long list of benefits for our health.

It protects the liver against toxins, fights free radicals, aids circulation, improves blood-vessel health, and has anti-cancer properties. Because curcumin has natural anti-inflammatory properties, many people use it to combat arthritis conditions. You can purchase it as a supplement or have it in your spice rack. Curry is a blend of spices that contains turmeric.

Many amazing studies have been done on the curcumin compound with Indian people because it is a staple of India's daily diet. On average the daily consumption is 1.5 grams to 2 grams per person. This is unique in terms of studies because there is rarely a food specifically linked to the culture of a single country. The overall cancer rates in the United States are two to three times higher than in India. The rate of colon/rectum cancer is about eight times higher in the US than India. Prostate cancer is a whopping twenty-one times higher in the US![29] Indian people have been shown in studies to have one of the lowest rates of Alzheimer's disease, five times lower than that of the West!

For amazing health benefits make sure you have turmeric in your spice rack and find ways to use it often.

Learn to use spices and herbs in a way that will benefit you, improve your health and make you feel more alive! Who doesn't want to feel more alive?

Glorious Greens

Whether you have a serious or chronic disease, or just want to improve your health, feel better, and have more energy, food can make a world of difference. I am motivated to take the extra time to prepare a meal because I know I will actually feel better, and it will contribute to my health.

Learn to use spices and herbs in a way that will benefit you, improve your health and make you feel more alive! Who doesn't want to feel more alive?

Greens are a super healing food. You can find them at the grocery store or the farmers' market. Buy them organic if you can. Greens in our diet have a tremendous ability to improve our health. There is a great variety of available greens. Some examples are leaf lettuce, broccoli, kale, asparagus, bok choy, and collard greens.

Greens contain chlorophyll, which provides essential vitamins and minerals and purifies the blood.

Here is a list of some of the great benefits of greens that will motivate you to make sure your family includes these in their daily eating:

- Inhibits cellular damage
- Provides subtle light energy
- Helps prevent cancer
- Promotes regularity
- Aids in intestinal flora
- Lifts the spirit and improves mood
- Improves gall bladder and kidney function

Here is my favorite way to cook greens:

- Add about 1 tablespoon of olive oil to fry pan and heat slightly over medium heat. Add 1 or 2 cloves of chopped garlic and heat until fragrant, only about a minute.

- Add red pepper flakes to taste (optional).

- Add chopped vegetables (broccoli, spinach, bok choy, etc.) and sauté for a minute or two.

- Add 1 or 2 tablespoons of water, depending on how many vegetables you have, and cover with lid.

- Cook until tender. Do not overcook. Sprinkle with salt and pepper.

CONCLUSION

Build Your Terrain

I NOTICE SOME OF MY PLANTS in my garden are not thriving like I would like. The most annoying problem is the munching of tender leaves by insects. Insects tend to attack less vigorous plants. I look at what the plant needs: more sunshine, more water, less water. A healthy plant is more likely to have a resistance to these pesky bugs. The soil is a vital factor in the health of a plant. Instead of spraying pesticides on the plants, I am working to build up the soil with compost. I also sprayed a natural insecticide soap to discourage bugs.

If the soil is healthy, the plant will be better able to resist disease.

The same holds true for our bodies. By building our bodies up with foods that are rich in important nutrients and engaging in physical activity, we can keep them strong and vibrant and better able to resist disease. The body is a huge system in equilibrium, and there are some basic needs it has to keep functioning in balance.

Science tells us that we all have cancer cells in our bodies. Just like a seed has the potential of an invasive weed to find favorable conditions and overtake the garden; we should do everything we can to avoid a single seed from flourishing.

We can also build our immune systems to help ward off the invaders like viruses and bacteria and aid our bodies in resisting many diseases.

Our bodies are the terrain.

What kind of terrain do we have?

Is it depleted or enriched?

Is it in balance or out of balance?

Increase the foods in your daily eating plan that studies have shown inhibit cancer cells. Here is a list of some of the cancer-fighting foods:[30]

- Onions
- Garlic
- Leeks
- Curry
- Turmeric
- Broccoli
- Dark chocolate (at least 70% cacao)
- Green Tea
- Celery
- Citrus fruits (oranges, lemons, limes)
- Berries
- Tomatoes
- Ginger
- Lettuce
- Shitake mushrooms
- Parsley
- Spinach

Let's build and fortify ourselves with scrumptious food that contains all the necessary nutrients and make lifestyle choices to help us achieve balanced health and gives us the best possible opportunity to maintain it.

About the Author

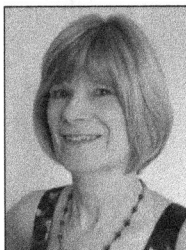

CAROL BEGAN HER JOURNEY as a certified Health Coach several years ago, but her introduction to the field of nutrition and wellness began decades before that. Over time, the connection between food, lifestyle, and health was apparent, and she found her energy and general health greatly improved.

She received her education from the Institute for Integrative Nutrition and has helped many people who are confused about what food choices to make or are struggling with health issues and don't know where to turn. Carol's many years of experience has yielded positive results in the people she has worked with.

Her clients have shown great improvement in many areas including, weight loss, digestive issues and in reducing or avoiding pharmaceutical solutions.

Carol is committed to showing people how to use food as a powerful means to create the greatest possible health for themselves. Everyone is different with varying needs, so the concept of bio individuality for each person is important to know about. Her emphasis is on working with others on finding ways to eat nutritious food and at the same time experiencing pleasure in eating. An integrative approach includes physical activity, stress reduction and finding joy in one's life. She listens carefully to what her client's goals are and works with them to achieve results.

> **For more information or to receive additional recipes contact Carol at:**
>
> *Create Health with Carol*
> carolcar@att.net
>
> www.CreateHealthwithCarol.com

End Notes

1. Bartoshuk, Linda. "Center for Smell and Taste." *Center for Smell and Taste*. N.p., n.d. Web. 02

2. Workman, Jennifer. *Stop Your Cravings: A Balanced Approach to Burning Fat, Increasing Energy, and Reducing Stress*. New York: Free, 2002. Print.

3. Stitt, Paul A. Beating the Food Giants. Manitowoc, WI: Natural, 1993. Print. pg. 120

4. Perlmutter, David, and Kristin Loberg. *Grain Brain: The Surprising Truth about Wheat, Carbs, and Sugar—your Brain's Silent Killers*. Little, Brown and Company, 2013. Print. Pg. 164

5. http://www.drjomd.com

6. "Obesity in Children." Centers for Disease Control and Prevention. Centers for Disease Control and Prevention, 06 Jan. 2015. Web. 12 Mar. 2015. http://www.cdc.gov/

7. "Insulin and Its Metabolic Effects." *Mercola.com*. Web. 12 Mar. 2015. <http://www.mercola.com/>.

8. Dufty, William. Sugar Blues. Radnor, PA: Chilton Book, 1975. Print. pg .22

9. Dufty, William. Sugar Blues. Radnor, PA: Chilton Book, 1975. Print. pg .23

10. Genzlinger, Kelly. Sugar-- Stop the Addiction: A Biochemical Explanation and Treatment Protocol for Healing from Refined Carbohydrate Dependency. Birmingham, MI: Holistic Hand, 2009. Print. pg.25

11. "Vegetables and Fruits: Get Plenty Every Day." The Nutrition Source. Web. 11 Mar. 2015. http://www.hsph.harvard.edu/nutritionsource/vegetables-full-story

12. Davis, William. *Wheat Belly: Lose the Wheat, Lose the Weight, and Find Your Path Back to Health.* Emmaus, Penn.: Rodale, 2011. Print. pg.221

13. Béliveau, Richard, and Denis Gingras. *Foods to Fight Cancer: Essential Foods to Help Prevent Cancer.* New York: DK Pub., 2007. Print.

14. Nestle, Marion. *Food Politics: How the Food Industry Influences Nutrition and Health.* Berkeley: U of California, 2002. Print. pg.38-42

15. Dadd-Redalia, Debra, Steve Lett, Judy Collins, and Debra Dadd-Redalia. Nontoxic, Natural & Earthwise: How to Protect Yourself and Your Family from Harmful Products and Live in Harmony with the Earth. Los Angeles: Jeremy P. Tarcher, 1990. Print. pg.148

16. Dadd-Redalia, Debra, Steve Lett, Judy Collins, and Debra Dadd-Redalia. Nontoxic, Natural & Earthwise: How to Protect Yourself and Your Family from Harmful Products and Live in Harmony with the Earth. Los Angeles: Jeremy P. Tarcher, 1990. Print. pg.150

17. www.safecosmetics.org

18. http://eartheasy.com/grow

19. Gedgaudas, Nora T. *Primal Body, Primal Mind: Beyond the Paleo Diet for Total Health and a Longer Life.* Rochester, VT: Healing Arts, 2011. Print.

20. Genzlinger, Kelly. *Sugar–Stop the Addiction: A Biochemical Explanation and Treatment Protocol for Healing from Refined Carbohydrate Dependency.* Birmingham, MI: Holistic Hand, 2009. Print. pg.74

21. "Seven County Study." Web. www.sevencountriesstudy.com.

22. Malhotra, Aseem. 22 Oct. 2013. Web.

23. "Seven Reasons to Eat More Saturated Fat." 22 Sept. 2009. Web.

24. Vanderhaeghe, Lorna R., and Karlene Karst. *Healthy Fats for Life: Preventing and Treating Common Health Problems with Essential Fatty Acids.* New York: Wiley, 2004. Print. pg.6

25. Fallon, Sally, Mary G. Enig, Kim Murray, and Marion Dearth. *Nourishing Traditions: The Cookbook That Challenges Politically Correct Nutrition and the Diet Dictocrats.* Brandywine, MD: NewTrends Pub., 2001. Print. pg.332

26. Perlmutter, David, and Kristin Loberg. *Grain Brain: The Surprising Truth about Wheat, Carbs, and Sugar--your Brain's Silent Killers.* Little, Brown and Company, 2013. Print.

27. Fallon, Sally, Mary G. Enig, Kim Murray, and Marion Dearth.

Nourishing Traditions: The Cookbook That Challenges Politically Correct Nutrition and the Diet Dictocrats. Brandywine, MD: NewTrends Pub., 2001. Print. pg.506

28. Fallon, Sally, Mary G. Enig, Kim Murray, and Marion Dearth. *Nourishing Traditions: The Cookbook That Challenges Politically Correct Nutrition and the Diet Dictocrats.* Brandywine, MD: NewTrends Pub., 2001. Print. pg.96

29. Béliveau, Richard, and Denis Gingras. *Foods to Fight Cancer: Essential Foods to Help Prevent Cancer.* New York: DK Pub., 2007. Print. pg.102

30. Béliveau, Richard, and Denis Gingras. *Foods to Fight Cancer: Essential Foods to Help Prevent Cancer.* New York: DK Pub., 2007. Print.

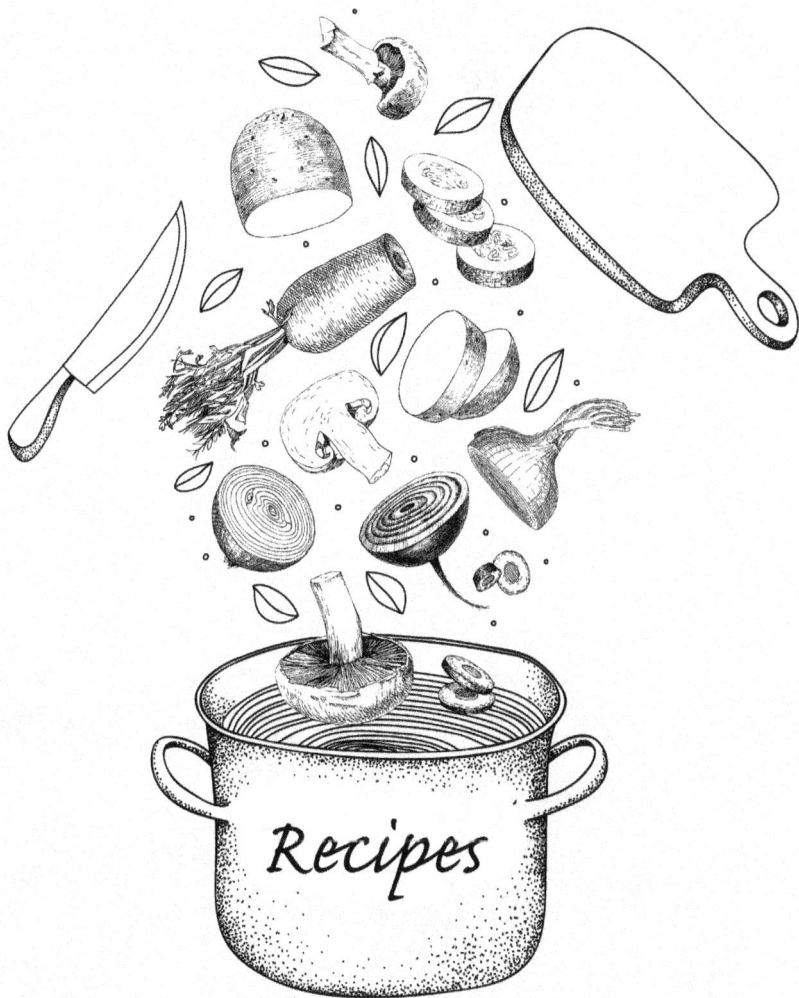

Recipes

Pecan French Toast

Serves 2

Sprouted grain bread is made by sprouting the seeds of the grain, drying them, and grinding them into a sort of "flour." By this processing, the digestibility of the grain is improved, the fiber is higher, and the glycemic index is lowered, which means the sugar is released slower in the bloodstream. You can purchase sprouted bread at a health food store or grocery store. The pecans in this become lightly toasted and give a nice flavor.

Ingredients

2 slices of sprouted multigrain bread

2 large eggs

2 tablespoons of milk or milk substitute (almond or coconut milk)

½ cup pecans or walnuts, chopped

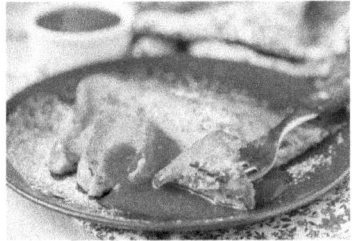

Directions

1. Beat eggs with milk in a shallow bowl. Immerse first slice of bread in egg mixture.
2. Soak for a minute or two and flip over and soak about another minute or two (using about half the egg mixture).
3. While the egg is soaking, heat fry pan to medium low heat and add small amount of oil or butter (about ½ teaspoon).
4. Place first slice in fry pan and sprinkle half the pecans on top of bread. Press pecans gently into bread with a spatula.
5. Take the second slice of bread and repeat the soaking process. Flip the first slice that is in the fry pan and cook the second side until firm. Remove from pan and keep warm. Repeat the cooking process for the second slice.
6. Serve with maple syrup, pear preserves, apple butter, or coconut cinnamon spread.

Coconut Cinnamon Spread

Ingredients

2 tablespoons coconut oil (It should be solid. If because of hot weather, it is liquid—put in refrigerator for a while until firm, but still soft.)

2 tablespoons soft butter

½ teaspoon raw honey

Sprinkle of cinnamon, to taste (approximately 1/8 teaspoon)

Directions

Mix all ingredients together until smooth.

~~~~~~~~~~~~~~~~~~

Orange Yogurt

Serves 2

Have this yogurt with your breakfast or as a snack. It is a good source of protein. It has sugar from the dates, but they contain natural sugar and fiber and won't rob nutrients from your body like refined sugars. Vitamin C, as we know, helps boost our immune system. Oranges and other citrus fruits are a great source of phytochemicals, which studies have shown to block tumor growth.

Ingredients

1 cup plain yogurt

2 dates, soaked in warm water for a half hour

1 ½ teaspoons raw honey or to taste

1 teaspoon fresh orange juice

¾ to 1 teaspoon grated orange zest or to taste

½ teaspoon pure vanilla extract

¼ cup chopped walnuts or pecans, optional

Directions

1. If yogurt is thin, place a paper towel in a strainer and add yogurt. Strain out whey for about a half hour.
2. Finely chop dates.
3. Mix yogurt with all the ingredients; adjust sweetness and orange zest to taste.
4. Top with chopped nuts if desired.

~~~~~~~~~~~~~~~~~~

Curry Egg Salad

Serves 1 or 2

If you like the taste of curry, here is a super easy recipe you could use for a lunch or snack.

Ingredients

2 hardboiled eggs

1 tablespoon of mayonnaise

¼ to ½ teaspoon curry powder

Salt and pepper to taste

Pinch cayenne pepper (optional)

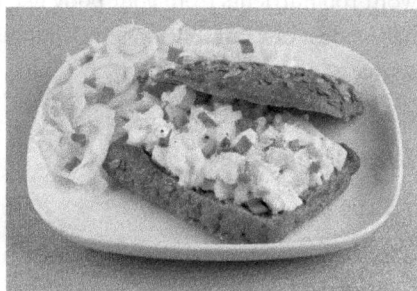

Directions

1. Mash eggs in a bowl.
2. Stir in other ingredients and serve on sprouted wheat or gluten free bread.

~~~~~~~~~~~~~~~~~

Veggie Wrap Sandwich

Serves 2

This is an easy, versatile sandwich. Try different veggies if you want, such as different kinds of peppers, a little chopped tomato, spinach or leaf lettuce in place of arugula. You can eat this sandwich at room temperature or keep the veggies warm before assembling sandwich.

Ingredients

2 or 3 teaspoons of olive oil or grape seed oil for sautéing vegetables

½ cup sliced red pepper

½ of a red onion, sliced

½ cup zucchini or yellow squash cut in about ¼-inch thick slices

1 cup arugula, coarsely chopped

½ cup fresh mozzarella cheese or other soft cheese (e.g., cream cheese, feta cheese)

Salt and pepper to taste

Whole grain sprouted tortillas

Directions

1. Heat a large skillet and add oil.
2. Add onion and cook for a couple minutes.
3. Add red pepper and continue cooking for about 2 minutes.
4. Add zucchini or yellow squash and cook until vegetables are tender. Set aside.
5. Heat tortillas by carefully holding them over a low-heat gas flame on stove, turning continually. You can also wrap in paper towel and heat in microwave.
6. Spread half of cheese mixture on each tortilla.
7. Divide the veggie mixture between the two tortillas. Add the amount of arugula you want and roll up tortilla. Enjoy!

~~~~~~~~~~~~~~~~

Mushroom Cheese Tortilla Roll

Serves 2

This is great for a light lunch or snack. Mushrooms have a lot of fiber and are a great immunity booster.

Ingredients

1 tablespoon butter or olive oil

¾ cup onions, thinly sliced

1 ½ cup mushroom, sliced (shitake, white button, or portabella)

¾ cup grated cheese (cheddar, gouda, or other)

2 tablespoons grated Parmesan (optional)

Salt and pepper to taste

4 tortillas (preferably sprouted wheat or corn)

Directions

1. Heat skillet and add oil.
2. Sauté onions on medium to medium high heat until golden.
3. Add mushrooms and black pepper and continue to cook until mushrooms are cooked through.
4. Carefully heat tortillas over low gas burner flame, turning continually. You can also wrap in paper towel and heat in microwave.
5. Spread ¼ of the hot-mushroom mixture on a tortilla and add ¼ of the grated cheese. Fold or roll to close. Repeat with each tortilla. Serve hot.

~~~~~~~~~~~~~~~~~~

Easy Tostados

Serves 4

Ingredients

1 tablespoon of olive oil

2 cups canned black beans or pinto beans, drained

1 medium onion chopped

1 medium green pepper, chopped

½ red pepper, chopped

2 cloves garlic, minced

½ teaspoon chili powder

½ teaspoon cumin

1 tomato, chopped or about 2 tablespoons of salsa

1 cup grated cheddar cheese

Salt and pepper to taste

Approximately 2 to 3 tablespoons water

4 sprouted tortillas (use sprouted corn for gluten free)

1 avocado, chopped (optional)

Sour cream (optional)

Directions

1. Heat olive oil in large skillet. Add onions and sauté about 2 minutes.
2. Stir in cumin, chili powder, salt, and pepper. Add garlic and cook until fragrant, 1 or 2 minutes.
3. Add peppers and continue cooking. Add tomato if using. Cook vegetables until soft, about 6 to 8 minutes.
4. Meanwhile preheat oven or use small toaster oven. Place tortillas on rack and heat until crisp.
5. Add beans to pan. Take a potato masher and gently mash the beans. Add a tablespoon at a time of water while mashing until the mixture is moist –not dry.
6. Spread bean mixture over each tortilla. Top with tomato or salsa and sour cream and avocado, if desired.

~~~~~~~~~~~~~~~~~

Red Beans and Rice

Serves 3 or 4

If you want a quick dinner or lunch, here is a vegetarian dish that is filling and satisfying.

Ingredients

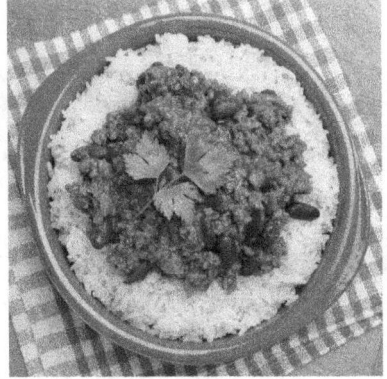

2 tablespoons olive oil

1 cup onion, chopped

1 cup celery, chopped

½ teaspoon cumin

¼ teaspoon mustard seed

½ teaspoon turmeric

2 cloves garlic, minced

1 16 ounce can kidney beans, drained

1 cup chopped tomato or canned diced tomato

1 to 2 cups vegetable broth

2 cups cooked brown rice

1 tablespoon chopped parsley

Salt and pepper to taste

Directions

1. Sauté onion in olive oil in a saucepan for a couple of minutes. Add cumin, mustard seed, and turmeric. Add celery and cook for a couple of minutes until tender.
2. Stir in garlic and cook until fragrant, about 2 minutes.
3. Add remaining ingredients, except parsley, and simmer together for about 20 minutes until flavors are blended. Sprinkle parsley on top and serve over rice.

~~~~~~~~~~~~~~~~~~

Grandma's Chicken Noodle Soup

Serves 8 to 10

Ingredients

1 whole chicken cut up
Extra package of chicken wings
3-4 celery stalks, cut into small pieces
2 carrots, sliced into small pieces
1-3 tomatoes (from a can)
1 large onion, quartered
4-5 sprigs of fresh parsley
1 bay leaf
4 whole cloves

1 tablespoon whole peppercorns
Salt to taste
32 ounce carton of organic chicken broth (optional to serve a larger group) 8 ounces flat, square egg noodles, boiled and drained or 1 ½ to 2 cups cooked brown rice
Parmesan cheese, shredded

Directions

1. Add all ingredients to a stock pot and fill to about two inches from the top with water.
   Let simmer for about two hours – skimming off any scummy foam that rises to the top.

2. Strain the broth into another pot or bowl and set chicken and veggies aside.

3. Cut the cooked chicken breasts into small shreds or pieces and return them to the stock along with as much celery and carrots you want in the broth. Use remaining chicken in another recipe such as chicken salad or a chicken stir fry.

4. Refrigerate the broth overnight and skim any fat off the top that rises to the surface overnight.

5. Reheat soup and add noodles or brown rice in the desired amount.

~~~~~~~~~~~~~~~~~~~

Curry Chicken Vegetable Soup

Serves 4

I was looking for a quick dinner one night and put this together in about 15 minutes. It was tasty and very satisfying on a cold winter evening. Make a vegetarian version by omitting chicken and adding 1 to 2 cups of beans.

Ingredients

1 to 2 tablespoons olive oil

1 medium onion, chopped

3 sticks celery, chopped

2 cloves of garlic, minced

1 cup mushrooms chopped

½ cup carrots, chopped small

½ cup diced tomatoes, fresh or canned

1 cup small cauliflower florets

1 cup broccoli florets

1 tablespoon tomato paste

1 ½ cups cooked chopped chicken (could substitute with chopped turkey, beef or beans)

32 ounces low-sodium, organic chicken broth or vegetable broth

1 cup water

1 ½ teaspoons curry powder (You could substitute with Italian spices such as basil, oregano and thyme.)

Salt to taste

¼ to ½ teaspoon crushed red pepper or to taste (optional)

Directions

1. Heat oil in large saucepan and add onions. Sauté for about 2 minutes.
2. Add celery and sauté for another 2 minutes.
3. Add garlic and stir and cook for about 1 minute until fragrant.
4. Add the rest of the ingredients, except the broccoli and mushrooms.
5. Simmer on medium heat for about 30 minutes, until vegetables are tender.
6. Add broccoli and mushrooms and cook for about 10 more minutes until done.
7. Taste and correct seasoning.

~~~~~~~~~~~~~~~~~

Senegal Fish Sauce

This is a nutrient-dense sauce. Ginger has a long list of benefits. It is a good source of zinc, an immune booster, and manganese, which helps in metabolism of fats and carbohydrates. Manganese is involved in the formation of bones and cartilage. Ginger fights inflammation, helps arthritis conditions, and stimulates circulation. Tomatoes contain lycopene, an anti-oxidant that studies have shown that it may hinder the development of cancer cells, prostate in particular. We can't forget garlic! It also has many health promoting properties: protects the liver and stomach, anti-bacterial, cleanses the colon, fights inflammations, and reduces cancer risk.

Ingredients

1 tablespoon olive oil

1 medium onion, chopped

2 to 3 cloves of garlic, minced

1 tablespoon fresh ginger, minced or grated

3 medium chopped tomatoes, fresh or canned

Juice of 2 limes

¼ to ½ tsp red pepper flakes or to taste

Salt and pepper to taste

Directions

1. Heat oil in large skillet. Add onion and sauté for a few minutes until soft.
2. Add garlic and cook until fragrant—1 or 2 minutes.
3. Add remaining ingredients and simmer for about 10 minutes. Add more tomato or water during the cooking process to increase volume if necessary.
4. Spoon sauce over grilled fish or chicken and enjoy.

Al's Salmon Grill

Serves 4

Ingredients

Marinade

1/3 cup soy sauce (Tamari is a naturally brewed soy sauce.)

2 tablespoons red pepper sauce like Franks

1 ½ to 2 lbs. fresh salmon fillet or steak cut

Lemon or lime slices

Directions

1. Trim and rinse fish fillets.
2. Mix soy sauce and red pepper sauce together.
3. Place fillets in glass casserole dish and pour marinade mixture over.
4. Place dish in refrigerator for at least an hour. Turn fillets over once.
5. Heat grill and oil the fish grill plate if using one.
6. If no grill plate, then oil the fish skin after blotting with paper towel.
7. Grill on high heat, skin side down 4 minutes per side. (5 minutes per side if steak cut, which are thicker.)
8. Before flipping brush some marinade sauce on top. Flip fish and continue cooking. Fish is done when flesh turns from translucent to opaque.
9. Remove from grill to a platter. Flesh side down, remove the skin by peeling off, then scrape away sub-skin gray matter with a paring or butter knife. Place finished fillets flesh side up on serving platter. Serve with lemon or lime slices.

Note: Under cooking fish on grill is easily adjusted. If translucent, put back on grill for additional 1-2 minutes. Once overcooked, no correction is possible. Gauging grill time is a matter of experience based on trial and error.

~~~~~~~~~~~~~~~~~~

Basic Stir-fry

Serves 4

Don't forget about a basic stir-fry for a delicious and quick dinner. If you want to save time, chop the vegetables and the meat ahead of time. I like to see what vegetables I have on hand already, so they don't go to waste. The cooking process will take about 10 to 15 minutes.

Ingredients

2 tablespoons olive or grape seed oil, divided

1 medium onion, chopped

2 or 3 cloves garlic, chopped

1 ½ to 2 cups of chopped veggies any combination (red or green bell pepper, broccoli, bok choy, spinach, zucchini, summer squash, cabbage, carrots, mushrooms, cut small so they will cook quickly)

1 ½ tablespoons soy sauce or tamari sauce (prefer wheat free)

1 to 1 ½ cups meat cut into ½-inch pieces (Substitute tempeh for protein.)

¼ to ½ cup water, chicken or beef broth

Red pepper flakes to taste approximately ¼ to ½ teaspoons

Directions

1. Heat large skillet and add 1 tablespoon oil. Add onion and sauté on medium high heat for about 2 minutes.
2. Add meat and brown lightly, about 2 minutes.
3. Remove meat and some of the onions from pan and set aside.
4. Add remaining oil to pan and add garlic, sauté for about a minute until it becomes fragrant.
5. Add chopped vegetables and cook on medium high heat, stirring almost constantly until tender crisp.
6. Add meat and onion back into pan. Add soy sauce and a little water. Cover and simmer for a couple of minutes.
7. Serve over brown rice, quinoa or whole grain buckwheat.

Note: If you like kimchi (a fermented Korean cabbage) add ¼ to ½ cup after this dish is done cooking. Kimchi is abundant in probiotics and fiber for a healthy gut.

~~~~~~~~~~~~~~~~~

Stuffed Peppers

Serves 4

Ingredients

2 medium to large green bell peppers or 3 poblano peppers

1 tablespoon of olive oil

1 medium onion, chopped

3 cloves garlic, minced

2 to 3 teaspoons cumin

1 lb. ground beef or ground turkey

2 to 3 tablespoons tomato paste

1 tablespoon cilantro chopped (optional)

Additional cilantro for sauce and topping

1 small green, red or orange pepper, chopped (optional)

1 small tomato, seeds removed, chopped (optional)

Salt and pepper to taste

1 to 2 cups cooked quinoa or rice (Filling should be moist but not too wet)

Directions

1. Preheat oven to 375 degrees. Cut peppers in half lengthwise, leaving the stem area intact. Cut out the ribbing and remove the seeds. Place the halves on a cookie sheet cut side down and bake for about 15 minutes. Remove from oven and cool.
2. Add oil to large skillet. Sauté onion until translucent. Add garlic and sauté for 1 or 2 minutes. Stir in the cumin spice. Add pepper if using and cook about 5 minutes. Add ground meat and cook until no longer pink. Add tomato, and tomato paste, salt and pepper. Cook on medium low heat for about 10 minutes. Stir in the cilantro if using and cooked rice or quinoa. Cook for a minute or two. Taste and adjust seasonings.
3. Fill pepper halves with filling. Place in 400 degree oven and heat--- about 15-20 minutes until heated through and peppers are tender.
4. Serve peppers with topping sauce and extra chopped cilantro, if desired.

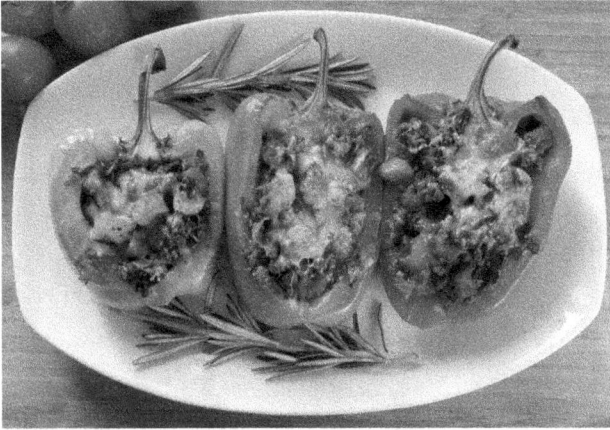

Sauce for topping peppers

Ingredients

½ cup sour cream

2 tablespoons cilantro or to taste

½ to 1 teaspoon lime juice

Directions

1. Blend or process all ingredients. Add a splash of water if too thick.
2. Taste and adjust to your preference.

~~~~~~~~~~~~~~~~~~

Mom's Chicken Cacciatore

Serves 4

Ingredients

1 tablespoons of olive oil (or 2 teaspoons of olive oil and 1 tablespoon butter)

4 chicken thighs

2 bone in chicken breasts with skin, halved crosswise (or your choice of combination of pieces)

1 large onion, chopped

1 large green pepper, chopped

2 or 3 cloves garlic, finely chopped

1 cup mushrooms, sliced (white button or baby portabella)

1 28 ounce can crushed tomatoes

4 to 6 ounces of dry red wine

Salt and pepper to taste

2 cups brown rice, whole grain buckwheat or quinoa

Directions

1. Heat saucepan and add oil/butter. Add chicken pieces and brown on both sides.
2. Take chicken out of pan and set aside.
3. Add onion and cook over medium heat for a couple of minutes. Add green pepper and continue cooking for 2 to 3 minutes. Add garlic and cook until fragrant—about a minute.
4. Add tomatoes, wine, salt and pepper. Return chicken to pan and simmer for 30-40 minutes until chicken is cooked through. Add mushrooms the last 15 minutes.
5. Take chicken out and when cool enough to handle, remove meat from bones.(optional) Place back in pan to heat before serving.
6. Serve over a whole grain such as brown or wild rice, buckwheat or quinoa.

~~~~~~~~~~~~~~~~~~

Fran's Kidney Bean Chili

Serves 6

This chili recipe is easy, satisfying, and full of fiber from the kidney beans, green pepper, and onions. It also provides a good amount of protein from the ground meat and beans.

Ingredients

2 tablespoons olive oil

1 medium to large onion chopped

2 cloves garlic, minced

1 medium or large green pepper chopped

1 pound of ground beef or ground turkey

1 15-ounce can red kidney beans, undrained

8- to 16-ounce can tomato sauce (depends how saucy you like it)

½ cup diced tomatoes, fresh or canned (optional)

1 tablespoon chili powder

Cayenne pepper or red pepper sauce (optional)

Salt and pepper to taste

Directions

1. Brown meat in oil in a large saucepan for a few minutes.
2. Add onion and sauté until soft (about 3 minutes).
3. Add garlic and cook until fragrant (1 or 2 minutes).
4. Add remaining ingredients and simmer over medium/low heat for about 1 hour, stirring occasionally.

~~~~~~~~~~~~~~~~~~~

Rosemary Potatoes

Serves 4

This is a great comfort food. Don't be afraid of the oil. Olive oil is a friendly fat, and our bodies need fat to burn fat. Fat also slows the release of sugar into your blood from the potatoes. Rosemary has a wonderful scent and taste and has great benefits. Here are few of them: fights free radicals, inflammation, bacteria and fungus, stimulates circulation and digestion, and acts as a decongestant. It also improves circulation to the brain, helps headaches, and helps lower high-blood pressure.

Ingredients

4 medium potatoes with skins

3 tablespoons olive oil

2 teaspoons dried rosemary, crushed with the back of a spoon or a mortar and pestle

Salt and pepper to taste

Directions

1. Scrub potatoes with a vegetable brush
2. Preheat oven to 500 degrees.
3. Cut potatoes in about 1 inch cubes.
4. Put potatoes in large baking dish or roasting pan.
5. Add olive oil and stir.
6. Add rosemary, salt, and pepper. Stir into mixture.
7. Bake for about 25 minutes. Check occasionally and stir. Be careful not to burn.
8. Place some folded paper towels in a bowl to absorb oil and remove potatoes with slotted spoon.

∼∼∼∼∼∼∼∼∼∼∼∼∼∼∼∼∼

Italian Vinaigrette Salad Dressing

Ingredients

2/3 cup olive oil

1/3 cup red wine vinegar or other vinegar

2 or 3 whole garlic cloves

¼ teaspoon dried basil

¼ teaspoon dried oregano

Salt and pepper to taste

Directions

1. Measure olive oil and vinegar into glass jar. Add garlic and spices.
2. Place lid on jar and shake.
3. Make ahead of time because the garlic will release its flavor into dressing.

This dressing will last a couple of weeks out of refrigerator. If the dressing has enough garlic flavor after a while, then remove garlic.

~~~~~~~~~~~~~~~~~~

Ginger Carrots

(Recipe from *Nourishing Traditions* by Sally Fallon)
This recipe is a great introduction to fermented vegetables. The sweetness of the carrots neutralizes the acidity that some people find disagreeable. Carrots are a rich source of carotenoids. Beta carotene, the most active form of carotenoids, has been shown to boost the immune system and to fight against cancer. Carrots also contain B vitamins, phosphorus, and calcium.

Ingredients

4 cups grated carrots, tightly packed

1 tablespoon freshly grated ginger

1 tablespoon sea salt

4 tablespoons whey, if not available, use additional 1 tablespoon salt

Take about 2 cups of yogurt and put it in a colander that you lined with a couple layers of paper towel. Place a bowl under the colander. The whey is what drips out of the solids of the yogurt.

Directions

1. In a bowl, mix all ingredients and pound with a wooden pounder or a meat hammer to release juices.
2. Place in a quart sized, wide-mouth Mason jar and press down firmly with a pounder or meat hammer until juices cover the carrots. The top of the carrots should be at least 1 inch below the top of the jar.
3. Cover tightly and leave at room temperature about 3 days before transferring to refrigerator.

~~~~~~~~~~~~~~~~~~

Sauerkraut

(Adapted from *Nourishing Traditions* by Sally Fallon)
Sauerkraut is a super food. It has lots of probiotics that will greatly benefit your digestion. It is high in vitamin C, B vitamins, and choline. Choline lowers blood pressure and regulates the passage of nutrients into the blood. It also aids the body in the metabolism of fats.

Ingredients

1 medium cabbage, cored and shredded

1 ½ tablespoons sea salt

4 tablespoons whey or an additional tablespoon salt

Take about 2 cups of yogurt and put it in a colander that you lined with a couple layers of paper towel. Place a bowl under the colander. The whey is what drips out of the solids of the yogurt.

Directions

1. In a bowl, mix cabbage, sea salt, and whey. Pound with a wooden pounder or a meat hammer for about 10 minutes to release juices.
2. Place in a quart-sized, wide-mouth jar and press down firmly with a pounder or meat hammer until juices come to the top of the cabbage. The top of the cabbage should be at least 1 inch below the top of the jar.
3. Cover tightly and keep at room temperature for 3 to 4 days before transferring to refrigerator. The sauerkraut can be eaten immediately, but it improves with age.

Cranberry Apple Crisp

Serves 8

This recipe is inspired from Jane Brody's recipe collection. It has a wonderful contrast of sweetness from the apple, tartness from the cranberries, and the color is irresistible. Instead of refined white sugar, I used dates to sweeten and add additional fiber. They contain iron, which helps carry oxygen to your cells. Dates contain potassium, which benefits your heart, and vitamin A, which benefits your eyes. Cranberries are super nutritious, because they are high in anti-oxidants—they could help prevent heart disease and are well known for treating urinary tract infections.

Ingredients

3 cups fresh cranberries (1 12-ounce package)

2 large apples, unpeeled, cored, and sliced thin

6 dates with pits removed (soaked in water for about a half hour)

1 teaspoon cinnamon

¼ cup almond flour, divided (found at a health food store or health section of the grocery store)

2 tablespoons of coconut flour (same place you will find almond flour)

¾ cup rolled oats (regular or quick)

½ cup chopped walnuts or pecans (optional)

3 tablespoons butter, melted

Directions

1. Drain water from dates and finely chop them.
2. In a large bowl, combine the cranberries, apples, dates, cinnamon, and 1 tablespoons of almond flour. Make sure the dates are evenly mixed through. Transfer the mixture to a greased, shallow baking dish.
3. In the same bowl, combine the remaining almond flour, coconut flour, oats and nuts, if desired. Stir in the melted butter and mix the ingredients well (the mixture should be crumbly). Sprinkle the oat mixture over the fruit mixture.
4. Bake the crisp in a preheated 375-degree oven for 40 minutes or until the crisp is lightly brown. Let the crisp stand for 10 minutes before serving.

~~~~~~~~~~~~~~~~~~

Maple Pecans

A handful of these pecans are satisfying if you want something sweet and crunchy. Pecans, like other nuts and seeds, contain healthy fats. There is a little sugar from the maple syrup, but it is a natural sugar and contains trace minerals. Grade B maple syrup has more minerals than grade A.

Ingredients

1 cup pecan halves

2 tablespoons maple syrup (the real stuff)

¼ teaspoon sea salt (unrefined —should be light grey or pink)

Directions

1. Put maple syrup in fry pan on medium heat.
2. Add pecans and sprinkle with the sea salt
3. As the pecans and maple syrup begin to heat up, stir constantly. The pecans will slowly absorb the syrup from the pan.

They are done when the syrup is absorbed and the nuts are mostly dry, about 10 minutes.

~~~~~~~~~~~~~~~~~

Sweetened Cacao Nibs

I make these occasionally as a treat. The cacao nibs are very bitter but the maple syrup adds some sweetness, and I like the crunch. A little of these goes a long way. They are good mixed with nuts and flaked coconut. Raw cacao, which is the raw ingredient in making chocolate, has been shown in studies to have four times the anti-oxidant effect of dark chocolate. It raises your serotonin levels, which is the mood hormone. Cacao also is very high in polyphenols, which are chemicals that have numerous health benefits, including lowering blood pressure and improving vascular function.

Ingredients

½ cup unsweetened cacao nibs (find at a health food store)

4 tablespoons maple syrup (the real stuff-preferably grade B)

Pinch of salt

Directions

1. Measure maple syrup into large fry pan. Spread the syrup out evenly. Sprinkle with salt.
2. Over low heat, stirring frequently, allow nibs to slowly absorb the maple syrup. This takes about 10 to 15 minutes.
3. Stir continually the last couple of minutes. The nibs are done when they are slightly crystalized and the pan is dry.

~~~~~~~~~~~~~~~~~

Chocolate Covered Strawberries

Makes 1 pint

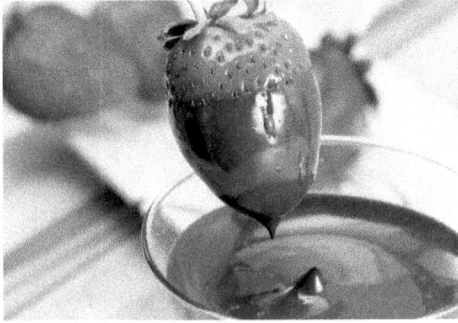

Ingredients

5 ounces dark chocolate, chopped (70 to 80% cacao content) If you are not used to dark chocolate start with a lower cacao content, maybe 60% and work your way up)

1 pint of strawberries with stems (preferably organic) Wash and allow to dry on clean dish towel.

Directions

1. Place the chopped chocolate in the top of a double boiler or a small saucepan set over a medium saucepan of simmering water. Stir occasionally until chocolate is smooth.
2. Holding berries by the stem, dip each one in melted chocolate, about three-quarters of the way up the stem. Place stem side down on wire rack and chill in refrigerator until hardened. Enjoy!

~~~~~~~~~~~~~~~~~